Praise for
ADHD Diagnosis and Management

"A friendly, inclusive guide to ADHD . . . Its great strength lies in its emphasis on how health professionals, educators, and families can best work together to optimize treatment."

—**Eugenia Chan, M.D., MPH**
Director, ADHD Program
Developmental Medicine Center
Children's Hospital Boston

"Provides a rare melding of information from the health and educational systems . . . an exceptional resource for clinicians and educators alike."

Christopher J. Kratochvil, M.D.
Chief Medical Officer, UNeHealth
Assistant Vice Chancellor for Clinical Research
University of Nebraska Medical Center, Omaha

"Sets a new standard for a comprehensive, up to date, scientifically sound desk reference and guide . . . must be on the shelf of every professional working with children with ADHD."

—**Sam Goldstein, Ph.D.**
Editor-in-Chief, *Journal of Attention Disorders*

"A valuable resource for understanding what is known about ADHD and using best practices for diagnosing and managing this disorder based upon scientific evidence."

—**Sandra Rief, M.A.**
Author, *How to Reach & Teach Children with ADD/ADHD* and *The ADD/ADHD Checklist*

"Highly informative, written in a direct, no-nonsense style, tightly linked to the available contemporary science, and guided by the decades of combined clinical experience of the authors, this is an exceptionally useful guide."

—**Russell A. Barkley, Ph.D.**
Clinical Professor of Psychiatry
Medical University of South Carolina, Charleston

D1598483

"Bridge[s] the knowledge gap between health care professionals and educators who both care for youth with ADHD . . . a very practical, innovative, and important book."

—**Mark A. Stein Ph.D.**
Director of ADHD Clinic and
Clinical Research Program
Professor of Psychiatry and Pediatrics
University of Illinois at Chicago

"Very well written, concise, comprehensive, practical, and highly useful."

—**Michael Reiff, M.D.**
Associate Professor of Pediatrics
and Family Medicine, University of Minnesota
Editor, *ADHD: A Complete and Authoritative Guide*

"Concise and packed with up-to-date information, a great resource for clinic-based and school-based professionals."

—**David L. Wodrich, Ph.D.**
Mary Emily Warner Associate Professor
School Psychology Program
Arizona State University

"Meticulously researched and accessibly written . . . should be required reading for any front-line professional who works with children with ADHD."

—**Michael Ching, M.D., MPH, FAAP**
Developmental Behavioral Pediatrician
Honolulu, Hawaii

"An outstanding resource for health care providers and educators . . . contains a veritable wealth of the latest evidence-based information for assessing and treating ADHD in clinics and schools and innovative methods for coordinating care across these systems."

—**Linda J. Pfiffner, Ph.D.**
Professor of Psychiatry
University of California, San Francisco

"A practical compendium of up-to-date research on assessment and treatment of ADHD. It is an invaluable reference for clinicians or educators who work with students with ADHD."

—**Robert Reid, Ph.D.**
University of Nebraska, Lincoln

ADHD Diagnosis
and Management

ADHD Diagnosis and Management

A Practical Guide
for the Clinic and the Classroom

by

Mark L. Wolraich, M.D.
University of Oklahoma
Health Sciences Center
Oklahoma City

and

George J. DuPaul, Ph.D.
Lehigh University
Bethlehem, Pennsylvania

Hartness Library
Vermont Technical College
One Main St.
Randolph Center, VT 05061

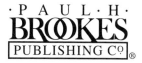

·P A U L·H·
BROOKES
PUBLISHING CO®

Baltimore • London • Sydney

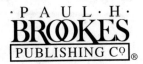

Paul H. Brookes Publishing Co.
Post Office Box 10624
Baltimore, Maryland 21285-0624
USA
www.brookespublishing.com

Copyright © 2010 by Paul H. Brookes Publishing Co., Inc.
All rights reserved.

"Paul H. Brookes Publishing Co." is a registered trademark
of Paul H. Brookes Publishing Co., Inc.

Typeset by Broad Books, Baltimore, Maryland.
Manufactured in the United States of America by
Versa Press. Inc., East Peoria, Illinois.

The information provided in this book is in no way meant to substitute for a medical or
mental health practitioner's advice or expert opinion. Readers should consult a health
or mental health professional if they are interested in more information. This book is
sold without warranties of any kind, express or implied, and the publisher and authors
disclaim any liability, loss, or damage caused by the contents of this book.

The individuals described in this book are real people whose situations are masked.
Names and identifying details have been changed to protect confidentiality.

Library of Congress Cataloging-in-Publication Data

ADHD diagnosis and management : a practical guide for the clinic and the classroom /
  by Mark L. Wolraich and George J. DuPaul.
      p.   ; cm.
  Includes bibliographical references and index.
  ISBN-13: 978-1-59857-035-9 (pbk.)
  ISBN-10: 1-59857-035-8 (pbk.)
  1. Attention-deficit hyperactivity disorder—Diagnosis.   2. Attention-deficit
hyperactivity disorder—Treatment.   I. DuPaul, George J.   II. Title.
  [DNLM: 1. Attention Deficit Disorder with Hyperactivity—diagnosis.   2. Attention
Deficit Disorder with Hyperactivity—therapy.   3. Adolescent.   4. Child.   5. Family
Relations.   6. Needs Assessment.   7. Schools.   8. Treatment Outcome. WS 350.8.A8
W866a 2010]
  RJ506.H9W655 2010
  618.92'8589—dc22   2010016801

British Library Cataloguing in Publication data are available from the British Library.

2014   2013   2012   2011   2010

10   9   8   7   6   5   4   3   2   1

Contents

About the Authors

Mark L. Wolraich, M.D., CMRI/Shaun Walters Professor of Pediatrics, Child Study Center, University of Oklahoma, 1100 N.E. 13th Street, Oklahoma City, Oklahoma 73117

Dr. Wolraich is Chief of the Section of Developmental and Behavioral Pediatrics at the University of Oklahoma Health Sciences Center. He received his M.D. from the State University of New York Upstate Medical Center in Syracuse. Dr. Wolraich completed a pediatric residency between Upstate Medical Center and the University of Oklahoma Health Sciences Center and completed a fellowship in developmental pediatrics at the University of Oregon Health Sciences Center. Dr. Wolraich has spent more than 30 years in research and clinical service related to attention-deficit/hyperactivity disorder (ADHD) and is a 2003 inductee in the Children and Adults with ADHD (CHADD) Hall of Fame. He has also been a major contributor to the development of guidelines for ADHD for primary care physicians by the American Academy of Pediatrics. Dr. Wolraich has been an author or coauthor on more than 150 journal articles and book chapters, including articles in the *New England Journal of Medicine, Pediatrics,* and the *Journal of the American Medical Association* and chapters in 20 books. His research is funded by the National Institutes of Health, National Institute of Mental Health, Maternal and Child Health Research Program; National Institute on Disabilities and Rehabilitation Research; the Centers for Disease Control and Prevention; and the Office of Special Education and Rehabilitation. Currently, he is investigating the prevalence and long-term outcomes of ADHD in five school districts.

George J. Dupaul, Ph.D., Professor of School Psychology and Chair, Department of Education and Human Services, Lehigh University, 111 Research Drive, Bethlehem, Pennsylvania 18015

Dr. DuPaul is Chairperson of the Department of Education and Human Services at Lehigh University. He received his Ph.D. in school psychology from the University of Rhode Island in 1985. Prior to his appointment at Lehigh, Dr. DuPaul was on the faculty at the University of Massachusetts Medical Center. He has extensive experience providing clinical services to children with attention-deficit/hyperactivity disorder (ADHD) and their families as well as consulting with a variety of school districts regarding the management of students with ADHD. He has been an author or coauthor on more than 160 journal articles and book chapters related to ADHD. He has published four books and two videos related to the assessment and treatment of ADHD. Dr. DuPaul serves on the editorial boards of several journals and is a former associate editor of the *School Psychology Review.* He is the recipient of the Senior Scientist Award from Division 16 (School Psychology) of the American Psychological Association and was named to the Children and Adults with ADHD (CHADD) Hall of Fame in 2008. Currently, he is investigating the effects of early intervention and school-based interventions for students with ADHD as well as the assessment and treatment of college students with ADHD.

Foreword

If you are reading this book, then you probably appreciate the serious difficulties associated with attention-deficit/hyperactivity disorder (ADHD) in terms of personal and societal costs. There have been studies published reporting the high financial cost associated with the impairment of individuals with ADHD and their treatment (e.g., Pelham, Foster, & Robb, 2007). In addition, there are data describing the adult outcomes of these youth, documenting the significant risks and challenges (Barkley, Murphy, & Fischer, 2008). There are also reports of the stress experienced by parents trying to help their children with ADHD succeed in spite of some difficult obstacles (Podolski & Nigg, 2001). Although the data are compelling, ultimately it comes down to individuals and their families.

The challenge is being face to face with a parent who is desperate to "save" his child from the path she is taking. Or the parent of an adolescent who is exhausted from years of efforts and is clinging to the hope that her child can still be helped. Or the adult who comes for assistance and reports a "run of bad luck" that, upon evaluation, appears to have existed his whole life. It is in the stories of individuals with ADHD that we can actually determine the progress we have made in caring for youth and adults with the disorder. Consider the stories of Jason, Tim, and Mike.

Jason

Jason was born a few weeks premature and was only a little over 5 pounds. He was the first born child of achievement-oriented parents, who thrust more hopes and dreams upon him at birth than is probably fair for any child. As a toddler, he was a very active child who ignored risk. He was constantly running and climbing and paid for it with a string of minor injuries. It seemed as if Jason was always happy, enjoying what he was doing and excited about what he was going to do next.

Although attending church and going to restaurants were difficult, his real problems began with the onset of school. Teachers in the early grades afforded him the extra attention he required, as he was a happy and cute boy who responded well to such attention. As he grew, being cute appeared to prove less salient to teachers and other adults who interacted with him. His parents were "invited" to chaperone field trips. Disruptive behavior and low levels of work completion were frequent problems that kept his teachers and parents in frequent communication, as they implemented a variety of behavioral interventions that kept him afloat through his elementary school years. Despite these challenges, Jason fared better than some because he was very social and well liked by most peers and adults.

Unfortunately, Jason began using drugs and alcohol toward the end of middle school and the beginning of high school. Jason continued to be well liked by peers and was frequently invited to parties and other social events. Discoveries of marijuana and alcohol at home led to Jason being grounded and receiving other restrictions. When he was in the ninth grade, and soon after completing a time period of being grounded, Jason was permitted to go to a party at a friend's house. The party was planned as a sleepover, but Jason was picked up at 11:00 by his parents because not all restrictions had been lifted. Later that night when everyone was asleep, the telephone rang, and Jason's father answered to hear a police officer ask if he was Jason's father. They had arrested Jason after they found him in a car that he had been driving with two passengers. Jason was not yet old enough to drive, had been drinking, and had stolen his father's car because he wanted to return to the party. After returning to the party in his father's car, to the cheers of his friends, he consumed more alcohol and then went driving with two friends. He turned a corner too fast and flipped the vehicle, sending it skidding on its roof down the middle of the road. One of the passengers was injured, but Jason and the other passenger were not.

Although Jason was suspended for a year for marijuana possession at high school, he ultimately graduated. He enrolled in community college, but poor grades and a lack of motivation led to his dropping out. He has worked as a cook and is returning to school in the culinary arts. Jason has been in a long-term stable relationship with a young lady he met in high school.

Tim

Tim, another child with ADHD, began participating in a school-based treatment program when he was in the first year of middle school.

Unlike Jason, Tim was very socially awkward and was frequently teased by peers. The bus rides to school, lunch in the cafeteria, and transitions between classes were particularly difficult for him. In spite of his regular victimization, he was usually smiling and eager to talk to anyone who would listen. In addition to receiving interventions targeting problems with organization, losing assignments, and not completing work, Tim received services focused on improving his social functioning. He reported enjoying participation in the program and attended 3 days per week; however, he was only minimally successful at generalizing gains made in the program to school and home.

During Tim's second year in the program, he told staff at the school-based program that he had finally found a group of friends with whom he could sit and enjoy lunch. The program staff, desperate for information confirming that he was making gains outside of the program, went to the cafeteria and observed Tim from a distance. Their high hopes came crashing down as they saw Tim get his food and then go to a table in the corner of the cafeteria reserved for students with disabilities from the self-contained special education classes. Tim sat at the table and began talking to the others while they looked at him occasionally, spoke to him once in awhile, and were content to let him sit there and talk to them. Cafeteria staff explained that although Tim had a history of not getting along with the other students, he had not been in trouble since sitting at that table. Staff from the after-school program left the cafeteria wondering about the definition of success for middle school students with ADHD and social impairment.

Mike

In middle school, Mike reluctantly began his participation in a Summer Treatment Program (Pelham & Hoza, 1996). He was diagnosed with ADHD at a young age. His parents reported an extensive history of problems interacting with peers and teachers, academic failure, and an unwillingness to abide by rules at home. They had tried to obtain help for him and their family from many sources, including his school, mental health professionals, and physicians, but nothing had proved to be very beneficial.

The Summer Treatment Program operated 9 hours per day, 5 days per week, for 8 weeks, and Mike attended every day. His behavior at the program was remarkably unlike his parents' description. He achieved better than most peers in the classroom, developed a leadership role within his group, and was one of the favorites of the staff. His parents experienced a remarkable combination of disbelief and excitement that increased with each occasion of feedback about Mike's progress. They participated in the parent meetings and reported progress at home, including improved relations with his siblings. One of the staff from the program continued to work with Mike and his parents during the academic year, and although Mike regressed compared to his behavior during the summer, he did experience some degree of success.

Mike returned the following summer to the program and continued his strong record of success. Following this second summer, however, Mike began experimenting with drugs and alcohol. His use was infrequent at first but increased, and as it did, his connection to his family deteriorated.

Mike's long-term outcome is unknown. His drug use continued to increase, and he began spending days in a row away from home. Ultimately, at 16 years of age, he never returned home, and his parents never learned of his whereabouts.

Treatment for Individuals with ADHD

As you read this book, I encourage you to think about Jason, Mike, and Tim, as well as the other individuals with ADHD whom you may know. The stories of these three individuals demonstrate that although we continue to make important progress in treatment development and evaluation for those with the disorder, there remains a lot that needs to be done. Current interventions for social impairment have resulted in limited success for most youth, and we are without reliable and valid tools to measure social functioning (especially with adolescents and adults). Effective prevention programs to keep children and adolescents with ADHD from using and abusing drugs and alcohol are sorely needed. In addition, effective assistance is needed for parents to cope with the increased monitoring, daily battles that seem endless and unnecessary, and the disasters that can change lives forever and tear families apart. Finally, it is important to note that all three of these boys were part of strong families with parents eager to do everything they could to help them. Most of our interventions are designed for families like these, but unfortunately, the consistent time, energy, and financial resources that the parents of all three boys expended on their children are not available to some families.

In this book, Drs. Wolraich and DuPaul blend together the science of treatment development and evaluation for individuals with ADHD and the realities of living with the disorder. They highlight the critical importance of partnerships and communication among youth, parents, educators, and health care professionals. The authors thoroughly review best practices and the science behind them but also discuss the application of these practices to the lives of the individuals we serve. I am not sure if the lives of Jason, Mike, and Tim would have been any different if the best practices described in this book would have been available when they were young, but I am confident that the best way to improve our science and practice of care is from the partnerships formed by parents, youth, practitioners, and scientists.

Steven W. Evans, Ph.D.
Professor of Psychology
Ohio University

References

Barkley, R.A., Murphy, K.R., & Fischer, M. (2008). *ADHD in adults: What the science says.* New York: The Guilford Press.

Pelham, W.E., Foster, E.M., & Robb, J.A. (2007). The economic impact of attention-deficit/hyperactivity disorder in children and adolescents. *Ambulatory Pediatrics, 7,* 121–131.

Pelham, W.E., & Hoza, B. (1996). Intensive treatment: A Summer Treatment Program for Children with ADHD. In E.D. Hibbs & P.S. Jensen (Eds.), *Psychosocial treatments for child and adolescent disorders: Empirically based strategies for clinical practice* (pp. 311–340). Washington: American Psychological Association.

Podolski, C., & Nigg, J.T. (2001). Parent stress and coping in relation to child ADHD severity and associated child disruptive behavior problems. *Journal of Clinical Child Psychology, 30,* 503–513.

Preface

Attention-deficit/hyperactivity disorder (ADHD) is a complex and challenging disorder. Despite extensive research covering the perspectives of psychiatry, psychology, education, pediatrics, speech and language, occupational therapy, and sociology, many questions remain unanswered. Even though extensive research has identified clearly efficacious treatments, the outcomes for many children with ADHD remain considerably less than optimal. A challenge presented by ADHD is that it affects multiple aspects of children's lives and requires input from multiple sources for its optimal treatment. It has a major impact on how children function in school as well as how they are able to interact with their peers and family. Thus, effective treatment of ADHD requires input from the health and mental health communities in addition to schools.

The need for communication and interaction between multiple systems, particularly health/mental health and education, is therefore a major consideration in the service issues that are essential to developing optimal management plans for children with ADHD. A first step in that process is ensuring that educators, physicians, and mental health workers are educated in the broader aspects of the diagnosis and treatment of ADHD within and across different systems. In this book, we have attempted to bring together those aspects through the coordinated efforts of authors who come from both the health and educational systems. The book provides essential information about both the diagnosis and treatment of ADHD in children in a language that is understandable to both clinicians and educators. We provide both perspectives so that those individuals who care for children with ADHD can understand the full scope of the issues and know how best to approach children with ADHD.

The organization of the book takes the reader through 1) the history of the condition and the extent to which it is present, 2) how schools can screen for the condition, 3) what diagnosis entails, 4) how to treat ADHD with both medical and behavioral interventions, and 5) what educational adaptations are likely to help children in the classroom.

We have based information on the scientific evidence available, while also utilizing our own experience in diagnosing and treating children with ADHD. References are provided to the extent possible for the information and recommendations included in the book. We have also recommended resources (see Chapter 11) that can be helpful to clinicians and school personnel in their interventions with children with ADHD. It is our hope that the book will help to provide a global perspective to the diagnosis and treatment process; help clinicians and educators to have a broader perspective about ADHD; and promote better communication among clinicians, educators, and families.

Acknowledgments

We wish to express our thanks to Kristen Carson, who helped with our literature searches.

To the DuPaul family,
wife, Judy, and sons, Jason and Glenn,
and the Wolraich grandchildren,
Ni-zhoni Palone and Simon Dolev

CHAPTER 1

Introduction and History

Attention-deficit hyperactivity disorder (ADHD) is a neurobiologic disorder manifested by inappropriate, inattentive, impulsive, and hyperactive behaviors that cause significant impairment. It is a condition that has been studied quite extensively, but despite all the information available, ADHD remains controversial, and people still question its existence. Manifestations of the disorder and services for children with ADHD span the general medical, mental health, and educational sectors and include both constitutional and environmental issues. Differences of opinion about the condition and its treatment are therefore not surprising. The extensive use or overuse of stimulant medication continues to be a publicized concern (Associated Press, 2009; Cohen, 2009; Cowart, 1988; Mayes, Bagwell, & Erkulwater, 2008). A great challenge to diagnosing and treating children with ADHD effectively is that it requires coordination between education and health/mental health providers. The impact of the condition and the interventions to treat it necessitate such coordination. The purpose of this book is to combine the important information from both educational and health/mental health perspectives to provide an integrated picture of the evidence regarding both the diagnosis and treatment across the health/mental health and educational systems.

Parents often have to be the sole communication link between their children's education and health providers. Some parents are able to take on this task very well but at the expense of an increase in their stress levels and demands for their time. Other parents may have found their own experiences as children with the health or education system to be daunting and have difficulty being the communication link their child needs. When direct information from the teacher is available, often there are discrepancies between the teacher's observations of the child's behavior and those of the parent because they observe the child in very different settings (Wolraich et al., 2004). Researchers in the Multimodal Treatment Study of Children with ADHD (Swanson, Conner, & Cantwell, 1999) documented the common discrepancies between parent and teacher observations and the apparent disconnect between educational and health services. They emphasized the importance of clinicians synthesizing their information about a child from both parents and teachers in making their decisions about diagnosis and treatment. The researchers further stated that information provided by the teachers is crucial to evaluate pharmacologic interventions. Teachers are in the best position to report on the efficacy and side effects of the medications because they observe children when medications are at peak levels (something which parents may not see).

Most physicians say they obtain teacher reports in their evaluation of children (Kwasman, Tinsley, & Lepper, 1995; Wolraich et al., 1990). However, one of the studies, which examined the agreement of physician diagnosis with the diagnosis based on teacher behavior rating scales, found agreement to be no more than 50%, whereas physician's diagnostic agreement with parents (obtained by structured interview) was 70% (Wolraich et al., 1990). This suggests that physicians get or weigh less information from teachers in their consideration of the diagnosis. The American Academy of Pediatrics (2000) made communication with both parents and teachers a major recommendation in its guidelines on ADHD and will likely maintain that recommendation in the forthcoming revised guidelines.

Fortunately, improvement in communication with parents was found in a subsequent survey of pediatricians (Wolraich, Bard, Stein, Rushton, & O'Connor, 2009). However, a number of difficulties remain with communication between physicians and teachers: They speak different languages. Both have jargon that facilitates their intraprofessional communication but makes interprofessional communication more difficult. They run on different schedules so that the times when teachers are able to communicate are frequently not convenient for physicians. Finally, they receive no additional compensation for the time required to communicate. E-mail has enhanced the possibility for communication, but its use is limited due to privacy restrictions.

Further complicating the issue of communication between parents, teachers, and physicians is the fact that, with each passing year, parents must often educate another teacher or set of teachers about their child's disorder and recreate channels of communication (Reid, Hertzog, & Snyder, 1996). Because active coordination is such a vital component of the diagnosis and management of ADHD, improving the amount of communication between the caregivers of children with ADHD is an area that warrants attention. The first step in such a process is educating teachers and health/mental health providers about ADHD, while considering education and health/mental health issues to provide an integrated picture.

History

Although ADHD seems to be a new and changing condition, particularly because of its recent identification as a disorder affecting adults, ADHD actually has a long history and has been of interest to a number of professional groups. In the mid-19th century, the characteristics of ADHD were represented by Heinrich Hoffman (1848), a German physician, by two characters, Fidgety Philip and Johnny Head-in Air, in his children's book (see Figure 1.1).

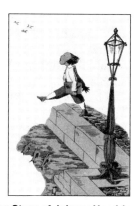

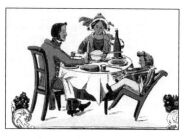

The Story of Fidgety Philip

"Let me see if Philip can
Be a little gentleman;
Let me see if he is able
To sit still for once at table":
Thus Papa bade Phil behave;
And Mamma looked very grave.
But fidgety Phil,
He won't sit still;
He wriggles,
And giggles,
And then, I declare,
Swings backwards and forwards,
And tilts up his chair,
Just like any rocking horse—
"Philip! I am getting cross!"

The Story of Johnny Head-in-Air

As he trudged along to school,
It was always Johnny's rule
To be looking at the sky
And the clouds that floated by;
But what just before him lay,
In his way,
Johnny never thought about;
So that every one cried out
"Look at little Johnny there,
Little Johnny Head-in-Air!"

Figure 1.1. The characteristics of attention-deficit/hyperactivity disorder as described in the children's book by Heinrich Hoffman (1848).

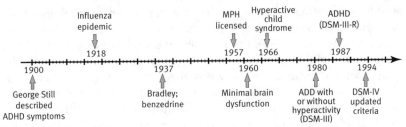

Figure 1.2. The history of attention-deficit/hyperactivity disorder (ADHD). (*Key:* ADD, attention deficit disorder; DSM, *Diagnostic and Statistical Manual of Mental Disorders*; MPH, methylphenidate.)

The timeline of the history of ADHD is presented in Figure 1.2. In 1902, at a meeting of the Royal College of Physicians, George Still described a disease he characterized as resulting from a defect in moral character. Still noted that the problem resulted in a child's inability to internalize rules and limits and additionally manifested itself in patterns of restless, inattentive, and overaroused behaviors. He suggested that the children had likely experienced brain damage but that the behavior could also arise from hereditary and environmental factors (Still, 1902).

The possible connection of ADHD to brain damage became more prominent in 1917–1918 following a worldwide epidemic of influenza with encephalitis. Some recovering children had symptoms of restlessness, inattention, impulsivity, easy arousability, and hyperactivity (Ebaugh, 1923; Hohman, 1922). In later years, many cases were seen with similar but less severe behavioral manifestations and no clear evidence of brain damage. As a result, the name of the disorder was changed to *minimal cerebral/brain dysfunction/damage,* or MBD (Clements, 1966).

For most cases of MBD, however, it was difficult to establish that the cause was brain damage. Therefore, the name of the condition shifted to one with less etiologic implications. As an example, based on the definition of the condition in the psychiatric classification system published in the second edition of the *Diagnostic and Statistical Manual of Mental Disorders* (*DSM-II;* American Psychiatric Association [APA], 1967), it was referred to as *hyperkinetic impulse disorder.* Later, because of the work of Virginia Douglas and others (Douglas, 1974; Douglas & Peters, 1979), the focus again shifted. The primary problem was considered to be inattention rather than hyperactivity, as reflected in the shift of the diagnostic label to *attention deficit disorder* in *DSM-III* (APA, 1980). The definition described the three broad behavioral dimensions of inattention, impulsivity, and hyperactivity. Two subtypes were defined: attention deficit disorder consisting of inattention and impulsivity and attention deficit disorder with hyperactivity that included all three dimensions. However, in the *DSM-III-R* (APA, 1987), the three dimensions were recombined into only one subtype: attention-deficit/hyperactivity disorder. In the *DSM-IV-TR* (APA, 2000), because of increased evidence and consensus, hyperactivity and impulsivity were combined into one of the now two dimensions, and three subtypes were defined: inattentive, hyperactive/impulsive, and combined subtypes. Repeat studies have found hyperactivity and impulsivity to occur together (Wolraich et al., 2003).

Characterizing the heterogeneity of the disorder began with the change in focus to inattention as the primary deficit in *DSM-III*. Under this definition, two subtypes were defined: attention deficit disorder with and without hyperactivity. However, by the publication of the *DSM-III-R,* the impression was that there was not enough evidence to support the subtypes. Subsequent research (Lahey & Carlson, 1991, 1994) provided evidence so that *DSM-IV* (APA, 1994) included three subtypes. There has been some concern that the differences between inattention and hyperactivity define separate disorders rather than subtypes of the same disorder (Loney & Milich, 1982). The argument is that inattention is more of a cognitive or learning disorder, whereas hyperactivity is more of a disruptive behavior disorder. However, the distinctions currently do not change the therapeutic plan.

In addition to helping to shift the focus to inattention as the primary deficit, psychiatry also was the first clinical discipline to report the benefits of stimulant medication (Bradley, 1937), starting with Benzedrine and focusing on children in inpatient residential care. There was little activity subsequent to Bradley's work until the 1950s, when clinicians rediscovered his work and methylphenidate was released for commercial use in 1957. The use of stimulants specifically for MBD was boosted by reports of positive effects in both the psychiatric and pediatric literature (Eisenberg, 1966; Laufer & Denhoff, 1957; Laufer, Denhoff, & Solomons, 1957).

Educational interest in this condition began in the 1940s and 1950s with the problem of educating children with "organic brain damage." Strauss and Werner started with a series of studies comparing children with brain injuries to children with intellectual disabilities (Strauss, 1941, 1944; Strauss & Werner, 1941, 1943). They also developed educational interventions, such as intersensory integration training, the use of concrete objects to teach abstract concepts, and the removal of distracting stimuli from the classroom (Strauss & Kephart, 1955). Although their studies primarily addressed children with brain injuries, they also included children with similar but milder patterns of deficits who had no definitive evidence of brain injuries—children fitting the description of MBD.

The education community has continued to contribute significantly to the services provided to children with ADHD. Under the Individuals with Disabilities Education Act of 1990 (PL 101-476) and the Rehabilitation Act of 1973 (PL 93-112, Section 504 regulations), school systems have had to provide adaptations in the classroom and special education services if needed for children with ADHD. Although not as extensive as psychopharmacologic or behavioral modification studies, research has been undertaken to address specific school interventions (e.g., Shapiro, Dupaul, Bradley, & Bailey, 1996; Zentall & Dwyer, 1988; Zentall & Meyer, 1987). Some examples of school interventions are having clear and visible classroom rules (Paine, Radicchi, Rosellini, Deutchman, & Darch, 1983), providing task choices to students (Dunlap et al., 1994), and implementing a token reinforcement system (Pelham & Fabiano, 2008). These interventions are discussed in more detail in Chapter 8.

Although ADHD was originally identified in the 1800s and treatment with stimulant medications has been found to be effective, the public controversies continue to focus on the existence of the condition and the extensive use of stimulant medication. Concern about extensive use or overuse of stimulant medication was first raised in 1970. *The Washington Post* reported that 5%–10% of the children in the Omaha, Nebraska, school system were receiving stimulant medications to control their behavior. Although it was not substantiated and was felt to be an overestimate of the prevalence, the report led to a congressional investigation and was the impetus for further research about stimulant medications.

In the 1980s, the Church of Scientology's Citizens Commission on Human Rights questioned the existence of the diagnosis of ADHD and pushed for the banning of stimulant medications, emphasizing and exaggerating the potential side effects (Citizens Commission on Human Rights, 1987; Toufexis, 1989; Williams, 1988). The articles claimed that the medications were causing the children to be extremely passive and in a drugged state, had long-term severe side effects, and were causing children to become addicted. The harm caused by amphetamines when they are taken in the amounts used by individuals abusing the drugs were used to characterize the side effects seen in individuals taking the medication for ADHD, even though the evidence does not suggest that those individuals who take stimulant medication for ADHD are at greater risk for substance abuse because of the medication (Wilens, Faraone, Biederman, & Gunawardene, 2003). The publicity led to a decrease in the use of methylphenidate in the late 1980s (Safer & Krager, 1992). For example, the medication treatment rate in Baltimore County, Maryland, doubled every 4–7 years from 1971 to 1987, going from

1% in 1971, to 6% in 1987, and then dropped to 3% by 1991. However, there has been a considerable increase in the use of stimulant medications in the past 15 years. From 1991 to 1995, the rate in Baltimore County increased from 2.6% to 3.8% (Safer, Zito, & Fine, 1996) and there was as much as a sixfold increase in the production of stimulant medications (Drug Enforcement Administration, 1995), which led to further concerns about the excessive use of and rationale for stimulant treatment in both the scientific (Diller, 1996) and lay (Angier, 1994; McGinnis, 1997) literature. The increase was likely due to a combination of factors, including the development of newer long-acting formulations of stimulant medications and the findings that ADHD symptoms do not disappear with maturation for many individuals with ADHD as previously thought (Barkley, Murphy, & Fischer, 2007; Biederman, Mick, & Faraone, 2000).

Factors in the Study of ADHD

The controversy over the excessive use of stimulant medications relates to service issues and not to efficacy. The evidence over the years has clearly demonstrated that stimulant medications effectively reduce the core symptoms of ADHD, as described to a greater extent in Chapter 6 (Brown et al., 2005; Jensen et al., 2001). Therefore, most concerns raised about stimulant medications are about who gets treated rather than about the efficacy of the medications. The argument is that too many people are taking stimulant medications, with the implication that a number of people are being treated inappropriately (Diller, 1996). Although it is very difficult to ascertain who is being treated inappropriately, evidence indicates that a number of individuals with ADHD do not receive treatment (Jensen et al., 1999).

Although most of the controlled studies demonstrating the efficacy of stimulant medication (Greenhill, 1995; Miller et al., 1998; Swanson et al., 1993) have been performed in psychiatric or tertiary facilities (developmental-behavioral clinics or mental health centers), most stimulant medications are prescribed by primary care physicians. Pediatricians in particular provide the majority of the prescriptions (Rappley, Gardiner, Jetton, & Houang, 1995; Ruel & Hickey, 1992; Sherman & Hertzig, 1991). Primary care physician participation in the care of children with this disorder stems, in part, from the historical perception of ADHD as a biological rather than emotional condition and from the fact that pediatricians are generally the first health professional contacted by parents. In addition, primary care pediatricians usually have ongoing relationships with the children's families, so they are more likely to be the first asked for help.

Because of the high prevalence rates of ADHD, limited numbers of child psychiatrists, and increasing restrictions placed on mental health services in managed care, the treatment of children with ADHD will continue to require significant participation by primary care physicians. In addition, pediatricians will likely be the initial point of contact for a family because of the negative societal attitude toward mental illness. Society continues to perceive a mind–body duality even though scientific evidence has significantly blurred the distinction. Behavioral health services are compensated differently, often with more restrictions than general medical services, and most states have separate health and mental health departments. The managed care system continues to perpetuate this distinction through the development of behavioral health carveouts and pushes more children into the management of primary care physicians by limiting access to mental health services. For some parents, seeking psychiatric help for their children seems like an admission of poor parenting. These parents find it easier to consider ADHD as a neurologic condition, so they will usually seek help from their pediatrician or a child neurologist.

Because treatment for ADHD often takes place in primary care settings, it is important to study the services in that context. However, relatively little information is available. It is possible that the children treated in primary care settings are different from those involved in the efficacy studies. The children seen in primary care settings seem to be younger than those seen in psychiatric settings, with a greater likelihood of a co-occurring learning disability and fewer other comorbidities (Lindgren et al., 1990).

The different types of children cared for by primary care pediatricians reflect the heterogeneity in the condition and the imprecision in making the diagnosis. Despite its biological and familial origins, the diagnosis of ADHD remains dependent on behavioral observations (Baumgaertel & Wolraich, 1998). There are no pathognomonic measures to diagnose children with ADHD, despite attempts such as continuous performance tests (Corkum & Siegel, 1993) and neuroimaging (Zametkin et al., 1990) to objectively measure parameters of central nervous system functioning. The diagnosis of ADHD remains dependent on the observations of those adults most familiar with the children because ADHD is an externalizing condition; their observations are more valid than the reports of the children themselves (Lahey et al., 1987). The behaviors observed are also contextually dependent: The greater the need for concentration and the less interesting the stimulus, the harder it is for a child with ADHD to concentrate. As such, many of the behaviors manifest themselves more readily in the concentration-demanding setting of school, making teacher observation a major consideration in the diagnosis. Communication between physicians and teachers, although difficult, is therefore vital to the diagnosis and treatment of children with ADHD.

This book reviews the evidence available about the diagnosis and treatment of ADHD from both health/mental health and educational perspectives. It integrates these findings to provide a comprehensive understanding of the condition and how to treat it. It also discusses how to coordinate services across the sectors so that both health and educational providers can understand and integrate what they are able to provide into a broader system of care for children with ADHD.

References

American Academy of Pediatrics, Committee on Quality Improvement and Subcommittee on Attention-Deficit/Hyperactivity Disorder. (2000). Clinical practice guideline: Diagnosis and evaluation of the child with attention-deficit/hyperactivity disorder. *Pediatrics, 105,* 1158–1170.

American Psychiatric Association. (1967). *Diagnostic and statistical manual of mental disorders* (2nd ed.). Washington, DC: Author.

American Psychiatric Association. (1980). *Diagnostic and statistical manual of mental disorders* (3rd ed.). Washington, DC: Author.

American Psychiatric Association. (1987). *Diagnostic and statistical manual of mental disorders* (3rd ed., Rev.). Washington, DC: Author.

American Psychiatric Association. (1994). *Diagnostic and statistical manual of mental disorders* (4th ed.). Washington, DC: Author.

American Psychiatric Association. (2000). *Diagnostic and statistical manual of mental disorders* (4th ed., Text Rev.). Washington, DC: Author.

Angier, N. (1994, July 24). The debilitating malady called boyhood. *New York Times,* Sec. 4, pp. 1, 4.

Associated Press. (2009). *ADHD drug abuse calls flood poisons centers.* Retrieved November 23, 2009, from http://www.msnbc.msn.com/id/32538503/ns/health-kids_and_parenting/.

Barkley, R., Murphy, K., & Fischer, M. (2007). *ADHD in adults: What the science says.* New York: Guilford Press.

Baumgaertel, A., & Wolraich, M.L. (1998). Practice guideline for the diagnosis and management of attention deficit hyperactivity disorder. *Ambulatory Child Health, 4,* 45–58.

Biederman, J., Mick, E., & Faraone, S.V. (2000). Age-dependent decline of symptoms of attention deficit hyperactivity disorder: Impact of remission definition and symptom type. *American Journal of Psychiatry, 157,* 816–818.

Bradley C. (1937). The behavior of children receiving benzedrine. *American Journal of Psychiatry, 94,* 577–585.

Brown, R., Amler, R.W., Freeman, W.S., Perrin, J.M., Stein, M.T., Feldman, H.M., et al. (2005). Treatment of attention-deficit/hyperactivity disorder: Overview of the evidence. *Pediatrics, 115,* e749–e756.

Citizens Commission on Human Rights. (1987). *Ritalin: A warning for parents.* Los Angeles: Church of Scientology.

Clements, S.D. (1966). *Minimal brain dysfunction in children: Terminology and identification.* Washington, DC: U.S. Department of Health, Education and Welfare.

Cohen, E. (2009). *Does your child need ADHD drugs?* Retrieved November 23, 2009, from http://www.cnn.com/2009/HEALTH/07/30/adhd.drugs.children/index.html.

Corkum, P.V., & Siegel, L.S. (1993). Is the continuous performance task a valuable research tool for use with children with attention-deficit-hyperactivity disorder? *Journal of Child Psychology and Psychiatry, 34,* 1217–1239.

Cowart, V.S. (1988). The Ritalin controversy: What's made this drug's opponents hyperactive? *JAMA, 259(17),* 2521–2523.

Diller, L.H. (1996). The run on Ritalin: Attention deficit disorder and stimulant treatment in the 1990s. *Hastings Center Report, 26,* 12–18.

Douglas, V.I. (1974). Differences between normal and hyperkinetic children. In C. Conners (Ed.), *Clinical use of stimulant drugs in children* (pp. 12–23). Amsterdam: Excerpta Medica.

Douglas, V.I., & Peters, K.G. (1979). Toward a clearer definition of the attention deficit of hyperactive children. In G. Hale & M. Lewis (Eds.), *Attention and the development of cognitive skills.* New York: Plenum Press.

Drug Enforcement Administration. (1995). *Yearly aggregate production quotas.* Washington, DC: Drug Enforcement Administration, Office of Public Affairs.

Dunlap, G., dePerczel, M., Clarke, S., Wilson, D., Wright, S., White, R., et al. (1994). Choice making to promote adaptive behavior for students with emotional and behavioral challenges. *Journal of Applied Behavior Analysis, 27,* 505–551.

Ebaugh, F.G. (1923). Neuropsychiatric sequelae of acute epidemic encephalitis in children. *American Journal of Diseases of Children, 25,* 89–97.

Eisenberg, L. (1966). The management of the hyperkinetic child. *Developmental and Child Neurology, 8(5),* 593–598.

Greenhill, L.L. (1995). Attention-deficit hyperactivity disorder: The stimulants. *Child and Adolescent Psychiatry Clinics of North America, 4,* 123–168.

Hoffman, H. (1848). *Der Struwwelpeter.* Leipzig, Germany: Imsel Verlag.

Hohman, L.B. (1922). Post-encephalitic behavior disorder in children. *Johns Hopkins Hospital Bulletin, 33,* 372–375.

Individuals with Disabilities Education Act (IDEA) of 1990, PL 101-476, 20 U.S.C. §§ 1400 *et seq.*

Jensen, P., Hinshaw, S.P., Swanson, J.M., Greenhill, L.L., Conners, C.K., Arnold, L.E., et al. (2001). Findings from the NIMH multimodal treatment study of ADHD (MTA): Implications and applications for primary care providers. *Journal of Developmental and Behavioral Pediatrics, 22,* 60–73.

Jensen, P.S., Kettle, L., Roper, M.T., Sloan, M.T., Dulcan, M.K., Hoven, C., et al. (1999). Are stimulants overprescribed? Treatment of ADHD in four communities. *Journal of the American Academy of Child and Adolescent Psychiatry, 38,* 797–804.

Kwasman, A., Tinsley, B.J., & Lepper, H.S. (1995). Pediatricians' knowledge and attitudes concerning the diagnosis and treatment of attention deficit and hyperactivity disorders. A national survey approach. *Archives of Pediatric and Adolescent Medicine, 149,* 1211–1216.

Lahey, B., McBurnett, K., Piacentinit, J., Hartdagen, S., Walker, J., Frick, P., et al. (1987). Agreement of parent and teacher rating scales with comprehensive clinical assessments of attention deficit disorder with hyperactivity. *Journal of Psychological Behavioral Assessment, 9,* 429–439.

Lahey, B. B., & Carlson, C. L. (1991). Validity of the diagnostic category of Attention Deficit Disorder without Hyperactivity: A review of the literature. *Journal of Learning Disabilities, 24,* 110-120.

Lahey, B.B., & Carlson, C.L. (1994). Attention deficit disorder without hyperactivity: A review of research relevant to DSM-IV. In T.A. Widiger, A.J. Frances, H.A. Pincus, W. Davis & M. First (Eds.), *DSM-IV sourcebook* (Vol. 1). Washignton, DC: American Psychiatric Press.

Laufer, M., & Denhoff, E. (1957). Hyperkinetic behavior syndrome in children. *Journal of Pediatrics, 50,* 463–474.

Laufer, M., Denhoff, E., & Solomons, G. (1957). Hyperkinetic impulse disorder in children's behavior problems. *Psychosomatic Medicine, 19,* 38–49.

Lindgren, S., Wolraich, M.L., Stromquist, A., Davis, C., Milich, R., & Watson, D. (1990). *Diagnostic heterogeneity in attention deficit hyperactivity disorder.* Paper presented at the Fourth Annual NIMH International Research Conference on the Classification and Treatment of Mental Disorders in General Medical Settings, Bethesda, MD.

Loney, J., & Milich, R. (1982). Hyperactivity, inattention, and aggression in clinical practice. *Advances in Developmental and Behavioral Pediatrics, 3,* 113–147.

Mayes, R., Bagwell, C., & Erkulwater, J. (2008). ADHD and the rise in stimulant use among children. *Harvard Review of Psychiatry, 16,* 151–166.

McGinnis, J. (1997, September 18). Attention deficit disaster. *The Wall Street Journal,* p. A14.

Miller, A., Lee, S.K., Raina, P., Klassen, A., Zupanic, J., & Olsen, L. (1998). *A review of therapies for attention deficit/hyperactivity disorder.* Vancouver: Research Institute for Chilldren's and Women's Health and University of British Columbia.

Paine, S.C., Radicchi, J., Rosellini, L.C., Deutchman, L., & Darch, C.B. (1983). *Structuring your classroom for academic success.* Champaign, IL: Research Press.

Pelham, W., & Fabiano, G.A. (2008). Evidence-based psychosocial treatments for attention-deficit/hyperactivity disorder. *Journal of Clinical Child and Adolescent Psychology, 37,* 184–214.

Rappley, M.D., Gardiner, J.C., Jetton, J.R., & Houang, R.T. (1995). The use of methylphenidate in Michigan. *Archives of Pediatric and Adolescent Medicine, 149,* 675–679.

Rehabilitation Act of 1973, PL 93-112, 29 U.S.C. §§ 701 *et seq.*

Reid, R., Hertzog, M., & Snyder, M. (1996). Educating every teacher, every year: The public schools and parents of children with ADHD. *Seminars in Speech and Language, 17(1),* 73–90.

Ruel, J.M., & Hickey, P. (1992). Are too many children being treated with methylphenidate? *Canadian Journal of Psychiatry, 37,* 570–572.

Safer, D.J., Zito, J.M., & Fine, E.M. (1996). Increased methylphenidate usage for attention deficit disorder in the 1990's. *Pediatrics, 98,* 1084–1088.

Safer, D.J., & Krager, J.M. (1992). Effect of a media blitz and a threatened lawsuit on stimulant treatment. *Journal of the American Medical Association, 268,* 1004–1007.

Shapiro, E.S., Dupaul, G.J., Bradley, K.L., & Bailey, L.T. (1996). A school-based consultation program for service delivery to middle school students with attention-deficit/hyperactivity disorder. *Journal of Emotional and Behavioral Disorders, 4,* 73–81.

Sherman, M., & Hertzig, M.E. (1991). Prescribing practices of Ritalin: The Suffolk County, New York study. In L. Greenhill & B. Osman (Eds.), *Ritalin theory and patient management.* New York: M.A. Liebert.

Still, G.F. (1902). The Coulstonian lectures on some abnormal physical conditions in children. *Lancet, 1,* 1008–1012.

Strauss, A.A. (1941). The incidence of central nervous system involvement in higher grade moron children. *American Journal of Mental Deficiency, 45,* 548–554.

Strauss, A.A. (1944). Ways of thinking in brain-crippled deficient children. *American Journal of Psychiatry, 100,* 639–647.

Strauss, A.A., & Kephart, N.C. (1955). *Psychopathology and education of the brain-injured child* (Vol. 2). New York: Grune and Stratton.

Strauss, A.A., & Werner, H. (1941). The mental organization of the brain injured mentally defective child. *American Journal of Psychiatry, 97,* 1194–1202.

Strauss, A.A., & Werner, H. (1943). Comparative psychopathology on the brain-injured child and the traumatic brain-injured adult. *American Journal of Psychiatry, 99,* 835–838.

Swanson, J.M., Conner, D.F., & Cantwell, D. (1999). Ill-advised. *Journal of the American Academy of Child and Adolescent Psychiatry, 35,* 5.

Swanson, J.M., McBurnett, K., Wigal, T., Pfiffner, L.J., Lerner, M.A., & Williams, L. (1993). Effect of stimulant medication on children with attention deficit disorder: A "review of reviews." *The Council for Exceptional Children, 60(2),* 154–162.

Toufexis, A. (1989, January 16). Worries about overactive kids: Are too many youngsters being misdiagnosed and medicated? *Time,* 65.

Wilens, T., Faraone, S., Biederman, J., & Gunawardene, S. (2003). Does stimulant therapy of ADHD beget later substance abuse? A meta-analytic review of the literature. *Pediatrics, 111,* 179–185.

Williams, L. (1988, January 15). Parents and doctors fear growing misuse of drug used to treat hyperactive kids. *Wall Street Journal,* p. 10.

Wolraich, M.L., Bard, D.E., Stein, M.T., Rushton, J.L., & O'Connor, K.G. (2009, Aug. 25). Pediatricians' attitudes and practices on ADHD before and after the development of ADHD pediatric practice guidelines. *Journal of Attention Disorders.* (First published as doi:10.1177/1087054709344194 at http://jad .sagepub.com/pap.dtl)

Wolraich, M.L., Lambert, E.W., Baumgaertel, A., Garcia-Tornel, S., Feurer, I.D., Bickman, L., et al. (2003). Teachers' screening for attention deficit/ hyperactivity disorder: Comparing multinational samples on teacher ratings of ADHD. *Journal of Abnormal Child Psychology, 31(4),* 445–455.

Wolraich, M.L., Lambert, E.W., Bickman, L., Simmons, T., Doffing, M.A., & Worley, K.A. (2004). Assessing the impact of parent and teacher agreement on diagnosing ADHD. *Journal of Developmental and Behavioral Pediatrics, 25,* 41–47.

Wolraich, M.L., Lindgren, S., Stromquist, A., Milich, R., Davis, C., & Watson, D. (1990). Stimulant medication use by primary care physicians in the treatment of attention deficit hyperactivity disorder. *Pediatrics, 86,* 95–101.

Zametkin, A.J., Nordahl, T.E., Gross, M., King, A.C., Semple, W.E., Rumsey, J., et al. (1990). Cerebral glucose metabolism in adults with hyperactivity of childhood onset. *New England Journal of Medicine, 323,* 1361–1366.

Zentall, S.S., & Dwyer, A.M. (1988). Color effects on the imulsivity and activity of hyperactive children. *Journal of School Psychology, 27,* 165–174.

Zentall, S.S., & Meyer, M.J. (1987). Self-regulation of stimulation for ADD-H children during reading and vigilance task performance. *Journal of Abnormal Child Psychology, 15,* 519–536.

CHAPTER 2

Prevalence, Etiology, and Long-Term Outcomes

For children with attention-deficit/hyperactivity disorder (ADHD) to be identified and receive appropriate services, it is important to understand the scope of the problem: the number of children who have the condition, the frequency that other conditions co-occur with ADHD, and the likely long-term outcomes. This information is important for planning individual diagnostic and treatment services throughout a child's academic lifetime and for understanding the longer-term implications that the condition will have on the child's life. The extent of the condition also influences the planning and development of appropriate service systems to optimize the availability and effectiveness of treatment. It is also important for providers to know what happens to children who have ADHD when they grow up and the consequence of having co-occurring (comorbid) conditions. This information helps providers to educate families, develop an effective management plan, prevent secondary complications, and plan for the future. To address these issues, this chapter discusses the causes of ADHD, its frequency, associated conditions, and long-term outcomes.

Etiology

The origin of ADHD is not limited to one etiology (or cause) that can be easily identified with any blood test or brain image, nor are any neuropsychological tests able to provide the answer at this time. Multiple etiologies can manifest similar behavioral symptoms. As noted in Chapter 1, brain damage, such as prematurity or birth trauma, historically was thought to be the most common cause of ADHD, as reflected by the earlier name *minimal brain damage or dysfunction* (Clements, 1966). However, it has become clear that by far the most common cause is of genetic origin.

Genetics

The evidence for genetic etiologies does not follow a typical Mendelian pattern of a recessive or dominant single gene, but there are multiple studies that provide evidence for an underlying genetic cause:

1. Twin studies have found a heritability rate of 0.75, meaning that 75% of the variance in phenotype can be attributed to genetic factors (Barkley, 1998).

2. Family studies have also shown that adoptive relatives of children with ADHD are less likely to have the disorder than biological relatives (Alberts-Corush, Firestone, & Goodman, 1986; Morrison & Stewart, 1973).

3. Biological siblings have a 2–3 times greater risk of having ADHD than children without siblings who have ADHD (Biederman, Faraone, Keenan, Knee, & Tsuang, 1990).

4. First-degree relatives have a greater risk of having the disorder compared to controls (Biederman et al., 1990; Cantwell, 1972; Morrison & Stewart, 1971).

More specific associations with specific genes have been identified in a portion of individuals with ADHD. These are genes that help the production, release, reuptake, or metabolism of two of the neurotransmitters that appear to be associated with ADHD. They include the dopamine transporter gene (*DAT1*) (Elia & Devoto, 2007), the D4 receptor gene (Swanson et al., 1998), *DAT5* (Elia & Devoto, 2007), dopamine beta hydrolase (Elia & Devoto, 2007), norepinephrine transporter (Kim et al., 2008), synaptosomal associated protein (Elia & Devoto, 2007), and the human thyroid receptor gene (Hauser et al., 1993). There can be errors in the absence of the gene or repetitions of the gene or part of the gene that cause the gene to not function correctly.

The implications of the genetic etiology are that it is important to obtain a careful pedigree of family members. Relatives may not have been formally diagnosed when they were children; therefore, it is important to ask about behaviors and school performance rather than asking about only those who had been clinically diagnosed. It is not atypical to find that one or both parents have the same problem as their child. In addition, a parent with ADHD may find it difficult to adhere well to a therapeutic program (e.g., ensuring their child receives medication) or to provide the consistency required in an effective behavioral program. If school was a negative experience for the parents, they may be intimidated by their child's teachers and convey their negative attitude about school to their child. Professionals can help parents to identify the condition in themselves and seek treatment. Parents with ADHD are more likely to be able to follow through with the treatment plans for their children if they are being treated themselves.

Brain Injury

While genetic etiology is the most prevalent etiology, 20%–25% of individuals diagnosed with ADHD have their disorder associated with an organic (or physical) cause. Evidence for this finding can be found in the following studies:

1. A higher incidence of ADHD and learning disabilities among children who are born prematurely (Klebanov, Brooks-Gunn, & McCormick, 1994)

2. A higher incidence in children of women who smoke during their pregnancy (Fergusson, Horwood, & Lynskey, 1993)

3. Traumatic injuries to the brain, such as head injuries sustained in automobile or bicycle accidents, resulting in similar behaviors (Levin et al., 2007)

4. Exposures in utero, particularly to alcohol, causing ADHD symptomatology that, in its severe form, is manifested as fetal alcohol syndrome (Azuma & Cheshoff, 1993)

5. Exposure to substances such as lead (Needleman et al., 1979)

6. Infections such as meningitis (Shaywitz & Shaywitz, 1989)

Brain Mechanism

Regardless of the underlying cause, it is also clear that there are on average differences in both the size and function of certain areas of the brain in individuals with ADHD. Studies of brain anatomy in individuals with ADHD compared to those without ADHD based on magnetic resonance induction studies have demonstrated that, on average, individuals with ADHD have smaller brain sizes in prefrontal cortex, basal ganglia, and cerebellar vermix (Shaywitz, Fletcher, Pugh, Klorman, & Shaywitz, 1999). Complementing these studies, functional studies, such as positron emission tomography, single photon emission computed tomography, and functional magnetic resonance imaging, have shown decreased activity demonstrated by blood flow in the cordate area of the brain (striatal hypoperfusion) in individuals with ADHD compared to comparison individuals (Kelly, Margulies, & Castellanos, 2007). In addition, on a neurotransmitter level, it is clear that the functions important to ADHD relate to the dopamine and norepinephrine systems in the same areas of the brain identified by anatomical studies (see Figure 2.1). As neurotransmitters, both dopamine and norepinephrine are two of the chemicals that are released from the ends of a neuron and travel across the cleft between that neuron and the next neuron in the path that provides the communication among brain neurons and between the brain and nerve cells in the rest of the body. Although the differences in brain structures and function have been thought to be permanent differences, a recent

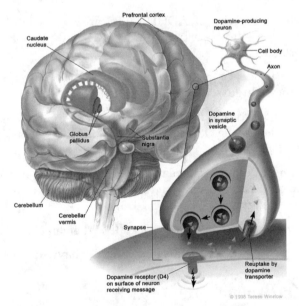

Figure 2.1. Neuroanatomy of attention-deficit/hyperactivity disorder. (Copyright © 1998 Terese Winslow. Reprinted by permission.)

longitudinal imaging study found that some of the differences between individuals with ADHD and a comparison group are due to delays in maturation, suggesting that they disappear in some individuals when they become adults (Kieling, Goncalves, Tannock, & Castellanos, 2008).

The differences in size and activity in the brain also are manifested in differences in neuropsychological functioning. These differences are found in what is described as *executive functioning.* Executive function skills can be thought of as the secretarial activities that help individuals function efficiently. They include the abilities to focus on one activity and filter out extraneous stimuli, to process information in working memory, to shift attention, and to regulate moods (Lawrence et al., 2004). People with poor working memories will have problems completing tasks, as well as difficulty paying attention and not being distracted.

Despite the advances in our understanding of the underlying differences and deficits in individuals with ADHD, the sophisticated assessment techniques that are now available, such as brain imaging, do not help to facilitate the clinical diagnosis. People with ADHD often have smaller and less active areas in the brain than people without ADHD, but there is a great deal of variation in both groups. These groups overlap so that the upper portion of the people with ADHD and the lower portion of the people without ADHD become indistinguishable. Neuropsychological tests do not consistently distinguish children with ADHD as independent measures and do not add information that is required to be able to diagnose children with ADHD. Therefore, despite the new research findings identifying the brain changes in structure and function, the diagnosis of ADHD remains dependent on the reports of those who most closely observe the children—parents and teachers. As with other mental disorders such as depression, schizophrenia, or anxiety disorders, the diagnosis is made based on the presence of specific behaviors or symptoms that occur for a defined amount of time and cause significant dysfunction. Like the aforementioned disorders, ADHD is a mental disorder with a significant biological basis for which some element of genetic transmission can also be found.

Prevalence

The prevalence of ADHD is a very important issue. It is at the heart of concern in the popular press that children are being overdiagnosed with ADHD and inappropriately treated with stimulant medications (Diller, 1996; Many Believe Drugs to Treat ADHD, 2006). Prevalence is also important information needed by both the health and education sectors in planning for the extent of services required. However, determining the true prevalence rate of ADHD has been a challenging task, as discussed in the following five issues.

First, there are no specific biological markers (laboratory tests or image studies) that can be used to establish a definitive diagnosis. As objective a measurement as possible is required to set a "gold standard." However, as stated previously, while the scientific evidence clearly shows the biological underpinning of the condition, the diagnosis is based on the presence of specific behaviors and dysfunction that are observed and reported by the child's caregivers. Therefore, the diagnosis must rely on the subjective judgment of these reporters as to the presence of the requisite behaviors and the extent of dysfunction. The judgments are made more subjective because there are no clear normative criteria about what frequency of any given behavior is normal for any given age. In contrast to assessing intelligence, for which there are clear normative guidelines for what tasks can be accomplished at any given age, the subjective judgment of the reporter is required in considering the inappropriateness of specific behaviors. Furthermore, these judgments are likely to be affected by the circumstances under which the individual is observed and the cultural norms of the situations and the observers. The criteria are made even more subjective by the lack of clear measures by which to assess dysfunction.

The second issue is that there is no clear demarcation between appropriate and inappropriate behaviors. For example, symptoms of hallucinations or delusions are clear manifestations of psychotic disorders that are not generally found in individuals who do not have some disorder. However, the behaviors in ADHD follow a more "normal" distribution, so some defined cutoff point has to be set in order to establish diagnostic criteria. For example, children may inappropriately get out of their seats, the frequency of which can vary depending on the circumstances; however, this only becomes significant if it is causing the child to get in trouble. Rating scales such as the ADHD Rating Scale IV (DuPaul, Power, Anastopolous, & Reid, 1998), the Vanderbilt Rating Scales (Wolraich, Hannah, Pinnock, Baumgaertel, & Brown, 1996), and the Conners Revised Rating Scale (Conners, Sitarenios, Parker, & Epstein, 1998) have tried to address the issue by providing normative data (e.g., frequency range for making careless mistakes with a large group of children), but the commonly used scales that are based on the *Diagnostic and Statistical Manual of Mental Disorders, Fourth Edition* (*DSM-IV*; American Psychiatric Association [APA], 1994) criteria only include the presence of negative behaviors. As a result, their distributions are not normative since the *DSM-IV* criteria used to make any diagnosis are not structured to be normatively based. The issue of the boundary line between what is normal and what constitutes ADHD is a prominent issue for both primary care physicians and teachers, who each deal with the full spectrum of children.

Third, most of the behaviors exhibited by children with ADHD are environmentally dependent. For example, children with ADHD may pay attention for an extended period of time when the stimulus is interesting to them, such as when playing a videogame, but they have difficulty maintaining attention for rote schoolwork. Capable parents learn to structure their child's environment to compensate for the child's deficits by providing a more structured and consistent setting. Likewise, teachers who run their classes with more explicit and consistent rules, are positive and reinforcing to children when they notice appropriate behaviors, and remain consistent are likely to have children with milder ADHD symptoms who are functioning better, thereby decreasing their impairment.

Fourth, the only practical method so far for determining the presence of the behaviors characteristic of ADHD and their impact, particularly in children, is by utilizing reports from parents and teachers, which frequently are in disagreement (Wolraich et al., 2004). The disagreement does not necessarily reflect inaccurate reporting. Teachers see children in situations that require a greater need to focus and pay attention because of the nature of the tasks and the fact that there is usually a much higher child-to-adult ratio than occurs at home. Thus, teachers may see manifestations that do not occur in the frequently less demanding situations of home. Teachers also have the advantage of having a much greater number of same-age peers under similar circumstances as a comparison group. On the other hand, teachers are not as likely to observe a child in as varied circumstances as parents are. The prevalence studies that use teacher ratings tend to find higher rates but usually do not include all the *DSM-IV* criteria. Parent reports of clinical diagnoses may underreport the true prevalence rate more than those based on parent-structured psychiatric interviews that are more comprehensive and systematic.

Finally, the criteria for diagnosing ADHD have changed over time. These changes have further complicated the process of determining the true prevalence of ADHD. The change from only one subtype in *DSM-III-R* (APA, 1987) to three subtypes in *DSM-IV* has increased the prevalence rate (Baumgaertel, Wolraich, & Dietrich, 1995; Wolraich et al., 1996). Initially, when brain damage was considered to be a primary etiology, what were described as "soft" neurologic signs were thought to be diagnostic of the condition. These neurologic signs may include delays in the abilities to distinguish right from left or to localize movements in one extremity, such as the hand, without having similar movements (overflow activity) in the other hand. The lack of skills such as those described above may be considered normal when present at an earlier age but are abnormal if their absence persists. These findings are now considered to be an indication of the poor coordination found in many children with ADHD but are not specific for the condition. As minimal brain dysfunction, the prevalence rate of such soft neurologic signs was estimated to be 5% (Minskoff, 1973). It increased in prevalence with the definition of ADHD in *DSM-III* (APA, 1980), in which two subtypes were defined. In addition, the requirement of inattention hyperactivity or impulsivity as diagnostic criteria when there was only one subtype resulted in a number of individuals not considered as having ADHD despite their difficulties with inattention and organizational skills. This older requirement excluded many females, who more frequently do not manifest hyperactive behavior. The prevalence rate has continued to increase despite the requirement in *DSM-IV* for the behaviors to be present in more than one setting. It was 3%–5% with *DSM-III* criteria, 4%–6% with *DSM-III-R*, and 8%–12% for *DSM-IV* (APA, 1994).

Because the diagnostic criteria have changed over time to conform to the conceptual changes, the prevalence rate ranges from 1% to 14% (Szatmari, Bremner, & Nagy, 1989), although it is usually quoted as 3%–5% (APA, 1994). Future changes in diagnostic criteria may cause a further increase in this rate. Within the same samples, the prevalence rates of ADHD increased from 2.6% for *DSM-III* to 6.1% for *DSM-III-R* (Lindgren et al., 1990), and from 9.6% to 17.8% (Baumgaertel, 1995) and 7.2% to 11.4% (Wolraich et al., 1996) from *DSM-III-R* to *DSM-IV*. However, caution must be taken regarding the last two studies because the new criteria require a degree of pervasiveness and impairment not determined in those studies. By adding the requirement for impairment, the rate decreased from 16.1% to 6.8%. A recent study of clinical cases reported by parents give a rate of 7.8% (Visser, Lesesne, & Perou, 2007).

Change in diagnostic criteria is not the only factor causing the variations in prevalence rates. Studies of prevalence rates are also dependent on the sample studied. The rates are different for samples from a mental health clinic, primary care, and community/school. Given these challenges, it is not surprising that there are varying rates. The prevalence rate has ranged from 4% to 12%, with a median of 5.8% (Brown et al., 2001). Rates are higher in community samples than school samples (10.3% vs. 6.9%), higher in males than females (9.2% vs.

3.0%), and higher with the changes in diagnostic criteria (*DSM-III* to *DSM-III-R* to *DSM-IV*).

Because ADHD has been identified and treated for close to 50 years, there are a number of individuals being treated with stimulant medication, which further complicates the determination of the prevalence rate. It is impossible to determine retrospectively if many of those individuals are accurately diagnosed and on effective treatment or inappropriately diagnosed and treated with medication.

Long-Term Outcomes

ADHD is not an inconsequential condition. Individuals with ADHD are at considerable risk of long-term problems, particularly if they do not receive treatment. Although it was originally believed that the condition resolved by puberty, it is now clear that the majority of individuals with ADHD will continue to manifest symptoms as adults (Ingram, Hechtman, & Morgenstern, 1999). ADHD symptoms remain problematic in approximately 66% of children with ADHD when they become adults. In approximately 40% of children with ADHD, symptoms continue to a clinically significant degree (Mannuzza & Klein, 2000). When compared to adults without ADHD, individuals with the disorder complete less schooling, hold less qualified jobs, have lower self-esteem, and have less adequate social skills. They are at greater risk for substance abuse, start smoking at a younger age, and have higher smoking rates (Hartsough & Lambert, 1987; Lambert & Harsough, 1998). Among individuals with substance abuse disorders, ADHD rates range between 15% and 25% (Schubiner et al., 2000; Wilens, 1998). ADHD is also associated with substance abuse of greater severity, including more frequent motor vehicle collisions related to substance abuse (Biederman et al., 1997; Schubiner et al., 2000).

Many individuals with ADHD who manifested hyperactive behaviors as children no longer manifest those behaviors as adults, although many still report sensations of restlessness. However, the manifestations of inattention and disorganization remain. Long-term follow-up studies of individuals with ADHD have found significant rates of poor academic outcomes, greater rates of legal difficulties, more difficulties with peer and marital relationships, greater rates of substance abuse, and greater rates of motor vehicular accidents and violations (Ingram et al., 1999).

References

Alberts-Corush, J., Firestone, P., & Goodman, J.T. (1986). Attention and impulsivity characteristics of the biological and adoptive parents of hyperactive and normal control children. *American Journal of Orthopsychiatry, 56,* 413–423.

American Psychiatric Association. (1980). *Diagnostic and statistical manual of mental disorders* (3rd ed.). Washington, DC: Author.

American Psychiatric Association. (1987). *Diagnostic and statistical manual of mental disorders* (3rd ed., Rev.). Washington, DC: Author.

American Psychiatric Association. (1994). *Diagnostic and statistical manual of mental disorders* (4th ed.). Washington, DC: Author.

Azuma, S., & Cheshoff, I.J. (1993). Outcome of children prenatally exposed to cocaine and other drugs: A pathanalysis of three-year data. *Pediatrics, 92,* 396–402.

Barkley, R. (1998). *Attention deficit hyperactivity disorder: A handbook for diagnosis and treatment.* New York: Guilford Press.

Baumgaertel, A., Wolraich, M.L., & Dietrich, M. (1995). Comparison of diagnostic criteria for attention deficit disorders in a German elementary school sample. *Journal of the American Academy of Child and Adolescent Psychiatry, 34,* 629–638.

Biederman, J., Faraone, S.V., Keenan, K., Knee, D., & Tsuang, M.T. (1990). Family-genetic and psychosocial risk factors in DSM-III attention deficit disorder. *Journal of the American Academy of Child and Adolescent Psychiatry, 29,* 526–533.

Biederman, J., Wilens, T., Mick, E., Faraone, S.V., Weber, W., Curtis, S., et al. (1997). Is ADHD a risk factor for psychoactive substance use disorders? Findings from a four-year prospective follow-up study. *Journal of the American Academy of Child and Adolescent Psychiatry, 36,* 21–29.

Brown, R., Freeman, W.S., Perrin, J.M., Stein, M.T., Amler, R.W., Feldman, H.M., et al. (2001). Prevalence and assessment of attention-deficit/hyperactivity disorder in primary care settings. *Pediatrics, 107,* e43.

Cantwell, D.P. (1972). Psychiatric illness in the families of hyperactive children. *Archives of General Psychiatry, 27,* 414–417.

Clements, S.D. (1966). *Minimal brain dysfunction in children: Terminology and identification.* Washington, DC: U.S. Department of Health, Education, and Welfare.

Conners, C.K., Sitarenios, G., Parker, J.D., & Epstein, J.N. (1998). Revision and restandardization of the Conners Teacher Rating Scale (CTRS-R): Factor structure, reliability, and criterion validity. *Journal of Abnormal Child Psychology, 26,* 279–291.

Diller, L.H. (1996). The run on Ritalin: Attention deficit disorder and stimulant treatment in the 1990s. *Hastings Center Report, 26,* 12–18.

DuPaul, G.J., Power, T.J., Anastopolous, A.D., & Reid, R. (1998). *ADHD Rating Scale IV: Checklists, norms, and clinical interpretations.* New York: Guilford Press.

Elia, J., & Devoto, M. (2007). ADHD genetics: 2007 update. *Current Psychiatry Reports, 9,* 434–439.

Fergusson, D., Horwood, L.J., & Lynskey, M.T. (1993). Maternal smoking before and after pregnancy: Effects on behavioral outcomes in middle childhood. *Pediatrics, 92,* 815–822.

Hartsough, C., & Lambert, N.M. (1987). Pattern and progression of drug use among hyperactives and controls: A prospective short-term longitudinal study. *Journal of Child Psychology and Psychiatry, 28,* 543–553.

Hauser, P., Zametkin, A.J., Martinez, P., Vitiello, B., Matochik, J.A., Mixson, A.J., et al. (1993). Attention deficit-hyperactivity disorder in people with generalized resistance to thyroid hormone. *New England Journal of Medicine, 328,* 992–1001.

Ingram, S., Hechtman, L., & Morgenstern, G. (1999). Outcome issues in ADHD: Adolescent and adult long-term outcome. *Mental Retardation and Developmental Disabilities Research Reviews, 5,* 243–250.

Kelly, A., Margulies, D.S., & Castellanos, F.X. (2007). Recent advances in structural and functional brain imaging studies of attention-deficit/hyperactivity disorder. *Current Psychiatry Reports, 9,* 401–407.

Kieling, C., Goncalves, R.R., Tannock, R., & Castellanos, F.X. (2008). Neurobiology of attention deficit hyperactivity disorder. *Child and Adolescent Psychiatric Clinics of North America, 2,* 285–307.

Kim, J., Biederman, J., McGrath, C.L., Doyle, A.E., Mick, E., & Fagerness, J., et al. (2008). Further evidence of association between two NET single-nucleotide polymorphisms with ADHD. *Molecular Psychiatry, 13,* 624–630.

Klebanov, P., Brooks-Gunn, J., & McCormick, M.C. (1994). Classroom behavior of very low birth weight elementary school children. *Pediatrics, 94,* 700–708.

Lambert, N.M., & Harsough, C.S. (1998). Prospective study of tobacco smoking and substance dependencies among samples of ADHD and non-ADHD participants. *Journal of Learning Disabilities, 31,* 533–544.

Lawrence, V., Houghton, S., Douglas, G., Durkin, K., Whiting, K., & Tannock, R. (2004). Executive function and ADHD: A comparison of children's performance during neuropsychological testing and real-world activities. *Journal of Attention Disorders, 7,* 137–149.

Levin, H., Hanten, G., Max, J., Li, X., Swank, P., Ewing-Cobbs, L., et al. (2007). Symptoms of attention-deficit/hyperactivity disorder following traumatic brain injury in children. *Journal of Developmental and Behavioral Pediatrics, 28,* 108–118.

Lindgren, S., Wolraich, M.L., Stromquist, A., Davis, C., Milich, R., & Watson, D. (1990). *Diagnostic heterogeneity in attention deficit hyperactivity disorder.* Presented at the Fourth Annual NIMH International Research Conference on the Classification and Treatment of Mental Disorders in General Medical Settings, Bethesda, MD.

Mannuzza, S., & Klein, R.G. (2000). Long-term prognosis in attention-deficit/hyperactivity disorder. *Child and Adolescent Psychiatric Clinics of North America, 9,* 711–726.

Many Believe Drugs to Treat ADHD Are Prescribed Too Often, Poll Finds. (2006, April 27). *The Wall Street Journal Online, 5*(7).

Minskoff, J. (1973). Minimal brain dysfunction: 3. Epidemiology. Differential approaches to prevalence estimates of learning disabilities. *Annals of the New York Academy of Sciences, 205,* 139–145.

Morrison, J.R., & Stewart, M.A. (1971). A family study of the hyperactive child syndrome. *Biologic Psychiatry, 3,* 189–195.

Morrison, J.R., & Stewart, M.A. (1973). The psychiatric status of the legal families of adopted hyperactive children. *Archives of General Psychiatry, 28,* 888–891.

Needleman, H., Gunnoe, C., Leviton, A., Reed, R., Peresie, H., Maher, C., et al. (1979). Deficits in psychological and classroom performance in children with elevated dentine lead levels. *New England Journal of Medicine, 300,* 689–695.

Schubiner, H., Tzelepis, A., Milberger, S., Lockhart, N., Kruger, M., Kelley, B.J., et al. (2000). Prevalence of attention deficit hyperactivity disorder and conduct disorder among substance abusers. *Journal of Clinical Psychiatry, 61,* 244–251.

Shaywitz, B.A., Fletcher, J.M., Pugh, K.R., Klorman, R., & Shaywitz, S.E. (1999). Progress in imaging attention deficit hyperactivity disorder. *Mental Retardation and Developmental Disabilities Research Reviews, 5,* 185–190.

Shaywitz, B.A., & Shaywitz, S.E. (1989). Learning disabilities and attention disorders. In K. Swaiman (Ed.), *Pediatric neurology: Principles and practice* (pp. 857–894). St. Louis: Mosby.

Swanson, J.M., Sunohara, G.A., Kennedy, J.L., Regino, R., Fineberg, E., Wigal, T., et al. (1998). Association of the dopamine receptor D4 (*DRD4*) gene with a refined phenotype of attention deficit-hyperactivity disorder (ADHD): A family-based approach. *Molecular Psychiatry, 3,* 38–41.

Szatmari, P., Bremner, R., & Nagy, J. (1989). Asperger's syndrome: A review of clinical features. *Canadian Journal of Psychiatry, 34,* 554–560.

Visser, S.N., Lesesne, C.A., & Perou, R. (2007). National estimates and factors associated with medication treatment for childhood attention-deficit/hyperactivity disorder. *Pediatrics, 119,* S99–S106.

Wilens, T. (1998). Alcohol and other drug use and attention deficit hyperactivity disorder. *Alcohol Health and Research World, 22,* 127–130.

Wolraich, M.L., Hannah, J.N., Pinnock, T.Y., Baumgaertel, A., & Brown, J. (1996). Comparison of diagnostic criteria for attention deficit hyperactivity disorder in a county-wide sample. *Journal of the American Academy of Child and Adolescent Psychiatry, 35,* 319–323.

Wolraich, M.L., Lambert, E.W., Bickman, L., Simmons, T., Doffing, M.A., & Worley, K.A.. (2004). Assessing the impact of parent and teacher agreement on diagnosing ADHD. *Journal of Developmental and Behavioral Pediatrics, 25,* 41–47.

CHAPTER 3

Screening Procedures

Children and adolescents with attention-deficit/hyperactivity disorder (ADHD) experience a variety of significant difficulties in home, school, and community settings as a function of their symptomatic behaviors. Furthermore, individuals with ADHD are at greater than average risk for development of other mental health or learning difficulties that require treatment (Barkley, 2006). As a result, it is important to identify children with ADHD as early as possible so that effective interventions can be implemented across settings. Thus, schools and outpatient clinics should use reliable and valid screening procedures to initiate the identification and intervention development process.

There are at least three possible situations where screening procedures should be implemented in clinic and school settings. First, universal screening can be conducted proactively to identify children and adolescents who may have significant ADHD symptoms. Second, individuals referred for evaluation due to behavioral or learning difficulties should be screened for possible ADHD, which would require additional assessment. Finally, screening can be done with children and adolescents with ADHD in order to identify whether additional behavioral or learning difficulties are present. Although assessment measures may be similar across contexts, each of these screening situations addresses different questions and leads to different outcomes. This chapter describes the screening procedures for each of these three situations. Screening procedures that are specific to outpatient clinic and school settings will be delineated. Particular attention is paid to the role of school personnel in the screening process given the myriad difficulties children with ADHD experience in educational settings. Finally, procedures and factors to consider in enhancing communication among families, schools, and community-based health providers in the screening process are discussed.

Universal Screening for ADHD

ADHD is a relatively common disruptive behavior disorder that is found in approximately 5% of the school-age population worldwide (Polanczyk, Silva de Lima, Horta, Biederman, & Rohde, 2007). The symptoms of ADHD typically lead to referrals to primary care physicians and other health care providers for treatment (Barkley, 2006). Despite the widespread recognition of this disorder and the apparent high probability for treatment referral, recent studies indicate that ADHD is relatively underidentified and undertreated in the general population. For example, Froehlich and colleagues (2007) examined the prevalence of ADHD symptoms in a large, epidemiological sample and found that only 48% of children who were reported to exhibit clinically significant levels of ADHD symptomatology actually had been diagnosed with the disorder. Of even greater concern, only 39% of these children were receiving medication treatment to address their symptoms. Undertreatment was particularly prevalent for children from lower socioeconomic backgrounds. Similarly, Pastor and Reuben (2008) found relatively low rates of service utilization in a large sample of children identified with ADHD, with only 14.6% receiving special education and 31.7% having contact with a mental health professional. Thus, health care and educational professionals should screen for ADHD in a proactive fashion to reduce underidentification and increase utilization of appropriate treatment services. There are two possible venues for universal screening: school/classroom and primary health care settings, each of which will be described in the following sections.

Schoolwide/Classwide Screening for ADHD

The school or classroom setting has several advantages as a location for universal screening of ADHD. First, because of compulsory education laws, all children (other than those who are homeschooled) attend public or private schools. Thus, this setting allows access to the child population that is not available in any other location. Second, certain aspects of classroom activity (e.g., the requirement to sit still and pay attention, as well as to complete effortful, independent tasks) frequently elicit ADHD-related behaviors. Therefore, the probability of detecting ADHD symptoms is increased. Finally, school-based screening can include both teachers and parents as informants, thereby enhancing the accuracy of identification given that parents and teachers provide unique information about child behavior in different settings and contexts (Essex et al., 2009).

Very few empirical studies have evaluated school-based, universal screening models for ADHD. One early study examined the Abbreviated Conners Teacher Rating Scale (Conners, 1969) as a screening tool in elementary school settings (Satin, Winsberg, Monetti, Sverd, & Foss, 1985). This brief measure was found to identify more than 90% of children meeting diagnostic criteria for ADHD in a school sample. Presumably, the lack of proposed screening models is due to the perceived high referral rate for children with this disorder and the concomitant assumption that because of the overt, disruptive nature of symptoms of this disorder, individuals with ADHD are unlikely to be overlooked. As discussed previously, however, epidemiological data suggest that a substantial percentage of the ADHD population has not been identified (i.e., diagnosed) and is not receiving appropriate treatment.

In the absence of established models for school-based universal screening, we propose a process as displayed in Figure 3.1. The first

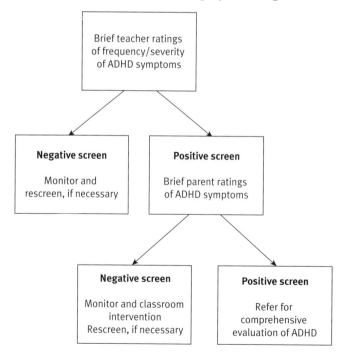

Figure 3.1. Model for school-based, universal screening of attention-deficit/hyperactivity disorder (ADHD).

Table 3.1.   Possible screening measures for attention-deficit/hyperactivity disorder (ADHD)

Measure	Citation	Respondent(s)
Vanderbilt Rating Scale	Wolraich, Feurer, Hannah, Baumgartel, and Pinnock (1998); Wolraich et al., (2003)	Parent and teacher
ADHD Rating Scale IV	DuPaul, Power, Anastopoulos, and Reid (1998)	Parent and teacher
ADHD Symptom Checklist 4	Gadow and Sprafkin (1997)	Parent and teacher
Disruptive Behavior Disorders Rating Scale	Pelham, Gnagy, Greenslade, and Milich (1992)	Parent and teacher
Swanson, Nolan, and Pelham Rating Scale	Swanson (1992)	Teacher

step in the screening process is collection of brief teacher ratings of the frequency and/or severity of ADHD symptoms. Several measures (see Table 3.1) are available for this purpose and take only a few minutes to complete. A cutoff score on the teacher rating should be established such that false negatives (i.e., children who have ADHD not identified by screening) are minimized as much as possible. (For more details, see Selecting a Cutoff Score for Screening Purposes later in this chapter.) For those students whose teacher ratings meet or exceed the cutoff score, the second step is to obtain parent ratings of the frequency and/or severity of ADHD symptoms. Once again, a cutoff score on the parent rating should be established such that false negatives are minimized.

The next step for those students whose parent ratings meet or exceed the cutoff score is a referral for a comprehensive evaluation of ADHD. As described in Chapter 4, this evaluation can be conducted in the school, primary health care, or mental health clinic setting and should include multiple measures across informants. The results of the comprehensive evaluation would lead to an accurate diagnosis and access to appropriate treatment services (e.g., medication, psychosocial treatment, academic intervention). For those students whose parent ratings did not meet or exceed the cutoff score, ongoing monitoring is recommended given high teacher ratings. A repeat screening may be conducted later in the school year to see if a comprehensive evaluation of ADHD is warranted.

Although this proposed model has not been subjected to empirical scrutiny, similar mental health and/or behavior disorder screening processes have been investigated. For example, Essex and colleagues (2009) designed a screening process for identifying kindergarten children who may be experiencing significant mental health difficulties associated with concurrent and later impairment. Parents and teachers of 328 children completed the MacArthur Health and Behavior Questionnaire (Boyce et al., 2002) during the kindergarten year. Children who exceeded established cutpoints for both externalizing (e.g., disruptive and aggressive) and internalizing (e.g., anxious and/or depressed) behavior difficulties showed stable symptoms throughout elementary school and were at significantly higher risk for academic and social impairment relative to their classmates. Of specific relevance to ADHD, students reported to exhibit externalizing problems were more likely to eventually show comorbid symptoms and impairment than those initially identified with internalizing problems. Based on these results, Essex and colleagues concluded that the early screening and intervention is necessary to address the chronic difficulties and impairment associated with mental health difficulties exhibited at school entry.

Bussing and colleagues (2008) obtained ratings on the Swanson, Nolan, and Pelham IV rating scale (SNAP-IV; Swanson, 1992) from parents and teachers of a randomly selected sample of 1,613 elementary school children. As was the case for the Essex and colleagues (2009) study, SNAP-IV ratings above a specified cutpoint were highly accurate in identifying students who met *Diagnostic and Statistical Manual of Mental Disorders, Fourth Edition* (*DSM-IV*; American Psychiatric Association [APA], 1994) criteria for ADHD in a subsequent comprehensive evaluation. The same study found that parent ratings were more accurate than teacher ratings in predicting ADHD diagnosis.

Walker and Severson (1988) devised the Systematic Screening for Behavior Disorders (SSBD) program for use in elementary schools. This screening process follows several stages or gates including 1) teacher nomination of students who exhibit the highest frequencies of externalizing and internalizing behaviors in the classroom, 2) completion of teacher ratings on a brief behavior problem questionnaire for student nominees, 3) direct observation of problematic behaviors for those students who exceed an established cutpoint on teacher ratings, and 4) referral for additional evaluation and intervention for those students whose observed behaviors are markedly aberrant in terms of frequency or severity. The SSBD is associated with positive outcomes in terms of accurate identification and successful treatment of those students who require services.

Screening for ADHD in Primary Health Care Settings

Universal screening for ADHD and related emotional or behavior difficulties can also be conducted in primary health care settings. As was the case for schools, no universal screening models specific to ADHD have been proposed and investigated for use in health care settings. However, models for broader-based screening of mental health problems have been described. For example, the American Academy of Pediatrics (AAP) Task Force on Mental Health (in press) will most likely recommend screening with the Pediatric Symptom Checklist (version with 17 or 35 items) (Gardner, Lucas, Kolko, & Campo, 2007; Jellinek et al., 1999) or the Strengths and Difficulties Questionnaire (Goodman, 2001) to identify children who require further evaluation of possible mental health difficulties.

Based on the AAP mental health task force recommendations, we propose a similar process of screening for ADHD as was described for schools. The first step should be to obtain parent ratings of ADHD symptoms, with those children whose scores meet or exceed an established cutpoint receiving additional screening. The next step should be to obtain teacher ratings, with those children whose scores meet or exceed the cutpoint being referred for a more comprehensive evaluation of ADHD as described in Chapter 4.

Selecting a Cutoff Score for Screening Purposes

Once rating scale scores are obtained, a decision must be made about whether further evaluation is necessary. The four statistical indices that aid in the selection of an optimal cutoff score for screening are sensitivity, specificity, positive predictive power (PPP), and negative predictive power (NPP) (see Table 3.2). Sensitivity represents the probability that children with a disorder (in this case, ADHD) are rated at or above a particular score. For example, if a score on an ADHD rating scale is associated with a sensitivity of 0.93, this means that 93% of children who are known to have ADHD score at or above this score. Sensitivity indicates the relative confidence a practitioner would have in generalizing from a disorder to a specific score or behavior.

Table 3.2.   Indices used to select screening cutoff scores

Index	Definition
Sensitivity	Probability that children who have attention-deficit/hyperactivity disorder (ADHD) receive a rating scale score at or above a particular cutoff score
Specificity	Probability that children without ADHD receive a rating scale score below a particular cutoff score
Positive predictive power (PPP)	Probability that a child has ADHD given a score at or above a specific cutoff score
Negative predictive power (NPP)	Probability that a child does not have ADHD given a score below a specific cutoff score

Specificity represents the probability that children who do not have a disorder (e.g., ADHD) are rated below a particular score on a rating scale. For example, if an obtained score is associated with a specificity of 0.90, then 90% of children without ADHD will score below this score. Similar to sensitivity, specificity represents the confidence a practitioner will have in generalizing from a disorder to a particular score or behavior. Sensitivity and specificity can range from 0 to 1.0 with higher scores (i.e., approaching 1.0) being preferred.

In contrast to sensitivity and specificity, PPP and NPP involve generalizing from individual scores or behaviors to a disorder. PPP refers to the probability that a child has a disorder (e.g., ADHD) given an obtained score at or above a specific threshold on a diagnostic index. For example, if the PPP associated with a particular rating scale score is 0.90, then 90% of children scoring at or above this cutpoint have ADHD. Conversely, NPP represents the probability that a child does not have ADHD given an obtained score below a specific threshold on a diagnostic index. For instance, if the NPP associated with a rating scale score is 0.92, then 92% of children scoring below this cutoff score do not have ADHD.

All four statistics can be used to help determine an optimal score for screening purposes. The relative priority as to which of the four statistics is most important will vary as a context of screening. In the case of schoolwide screening for ADHD in a general population, it is desirable to be as inclusive as possible because a subsequent comprehensive evaluation will provide more conclusive diagnostic information (DuPaul et al., 1998). In other words, one wants to minimize false negatives (i.e., children who have ADHD but are identified as not having ADHD) relative to false positives (i.e., children who do not have ADHD but are identified as having ADHD). Thus, a cutoff score that maximizes NPP and specificity is most useful in screening as this would enable practitioners to be highly accurate in predicting the absence of ADHD (NPP) and detect a relatively high percentage of children that truly do not have ADHD (specificity). Alternatively, when measures of ADHD are being collected as part of a comprehensive diagnostic evaluation, then practitioners typically want to be more exclusive given that the diagnosis of ADHD has implications for medication and school-based services. In this case, minimizing false positives takes precedence over false negatives. Thus, PPP and sensitivity become the most important statistics in setting a cutoff score, whereby the cutpoint should be highly accurate in predicting the presence of ADHD (PPP) and detect a relatively high percentage of children who truly have ADHD (sensitivity).

As an example of using these statistics to set cutoff scores for screening, Power, Andrews, and colleagues (1998) examined the NPP,

PPP, sensitivity, and specificity of various cutpoints on the ADHD Rating Scale IV (DuPaul et al., 1998) in a sample of 147 students in kindergarten to eighth grade in two public school districts. NPP was maximized using a cutoff score on teacher ratings that corresponded to the 80th percentile for children's age and gender. Theoretically, this cutoff score would identify the upper 20% of a given population for further assessment of ADHD. Although this is more inclusive than the estimated prevalence for this disorder (between 5% and 10%), the goal at the screening stage is to reduce the likelihood of false negatives because a more comprehensive evaluation emphasizing a reduction in false positives will follow.

Factors to Consider in Screening

Several factors should be considered when screening for ADHD in either school or primary health care settings. First, cutpoints on screening measures typically are set to minimize false negatives, assuming that the goal is to identify as many "true" cases of the disorder as possible. This means that false-positive identifications are likely in that some children who truly do not have ADHD will screen positive due to measurement error or other factors. Therefore, it is critical that a firm diagnostic decision is not made based on screening outcomes but on a comprehensive evaluation that minimizes false-positive identifications.

A second factor to consider when screening for ADHD is the degree to which age, gender, and ethnicity affect teacher and parent ratings of symptomatic behaviors. For example, Figures 3.2 and 3.3

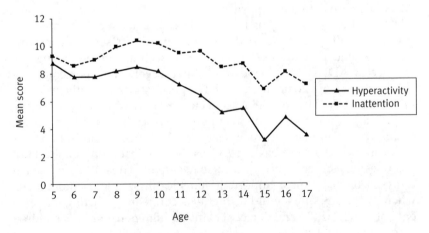

Figure 3.2.   Mean teacher ratings on the ADHD Rating Scale IV (DuPaul et al., 1998) for boys across age groups.

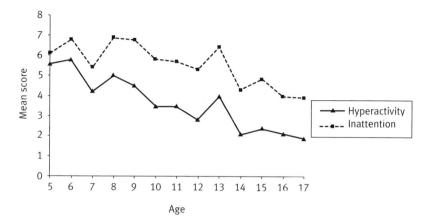

Figure 3.3. Mean teacher ratings on the ADHD Rating Scale IV (DuPaul et al., 1998) for girls across age groups.

show the relationship between age and teacher ratings for boys and girls, respectively. Data in these figures come from the standardization sample of the ADHD Rating Scale IV (DuPaul et al., 1998). In both figures, the mean rating for inattention and hyperactivity/ impulsivity diminishes across age, with younger children reported to exhibit these behaviors more frequently than adolescents. If one compares the data in Figures 3.2 and 3.3, it is also obvious that mean ratings for both behaviors are higher for boys than girls across the age span. These visually apparent age and gender differences are statistically significant and of relatively large magnitude (for details, see DuPaul et al., 1998).

Age and gender differences in the frequency of ADHD-related behaviors are well established and typically accounted for in the context of clinical assessments (i.e., by using standard scores or percentiles based on age and gender norms). However, another finding that usually is not accounted for in the screening or evaluation process is that teacher and parent ratings for African American children are significantly higher than those found for Caucasian children (Epstein, March, Conners, & Jackson, 1998; Reid, DuPaul, Power, Anastopoulos, & Riccio, 1998). For example, Figures 3.4 and 3.5 show mean teacher ratings across age and racial groups for inattention and hyperactivity/ impulsivity, respectively. In both cases, ratings are significantly higher for African American children relative to Caucasian children and, at some ages, are also higher than for Hispanic children. Thus, if cutpoints based on mixed race norms (i.e., primarily based on Caucasian children) are used, there may be a disproportional identification of African

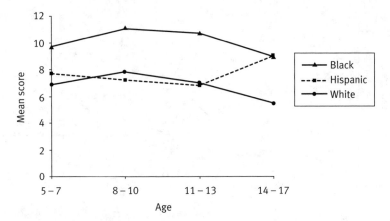

Figure 3.4. Mean teacher ratings of inattention on the ADHD Rating Scale IV (DuPaul et al., 1998) across ethnic and age groups.

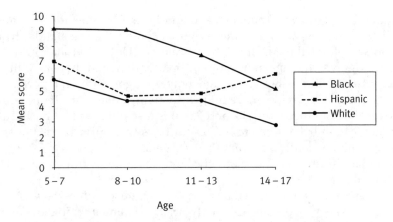

Figure 3.5. Mean teacher ratings of hyperactivity/impulsivity on the ADHD Rating Scale IV (DuPaul et al., 1998) across ethnic and age groups.

American children for further assessment. It is possible that future rating scales will account for this apparent ethnic group difference by using separate racial group norms; however, at present, clinicians must be cautious, particularly in situations where an African American child just meets or barely exceeds a rating scale cutpoint for ADHD.

A final factor to consider is that universal screening for ADHD is not currently a pervasive practice nor has much research been conducted on this topic. Although we have articulated solid reasons for why universal screening should be adopted, this process should be subjected to empirical scrutiny in applied settings before widespread adoption can be recommended.

Screening in Context of Multimethod Assessment of ADHD

Screening for ADHD should be conducted in any situation for which a child or adolescent is referred for evaluation because of attention problems, learning difficulties, or high levels of disruptive behavior. Furthermore, screening for ADHD should be conducted whenever a child is diagnosed with a disorder that is frequently comorbid with ADHD including conduct disorder, oppositional defiant disorder, an anxiety disorder, or a depressive disorder. In these contexts, screening should be considered the first step in the evaluation process. As an example of how screening is incorporated into a comprehensive evaluation, DuPaul and Stoner (2003) described a five-stage model for the school-based assessment of ADHD. The five stages include screening, multimethod assessment, interpretation of obtained data, treatment design and implementation, and treatment evaluation. In this context, screening is used to determine whether a comprehensive evaluation of ADHD should be conducted or whether ADHD does not appear to be a viable hypothesis for the child's difficulties. Therefore, evaluation should focus on other possible disorders.

Screening for ADHD at the individual level should be designed to answer two questions: Does the child or adolescent appear to exhibit clinically significant levels of inattention or hyperactivity/impulsivity? If so, is a comprehensive evaluation of ADHD warranted? Thus, screening procedures should be designed for cost and time efficiency while allowing for a certain degree of false-positive identifications. Stated differently, at this stage of the evaluation process it is better to err on the side of caution and identify those children and adolescents where there is at least a possibility of ADHD. At the same time, screening should eliminate from further consideration those individuals for whom the possibility of ADHD is relatively remote.

There are several methods that can be undertaken to screen for ADHD. One method is to ask a parent and/or teacher to complete a brief rating of ADHD symptoms. Several standardized, norm-referenced rating scales have been developed for this purpose including the Vanderbilt ADHD Rating Scale (Wolraich et al., 2003) and the ADHD Rating Scale IV (DuPaul et al., 1998). Both of these scales provide separate scores for inattention and hyperactivity/impulsivity symptoms. The respondent indicates the frequency with which each of the 18 symptoms of ADHD has been exhibited over a specific period of time (e.g., 6 months for parent ratings or 2 months for teacher ratings). Each item is rated for frequency on a Likert scale (e.g., ranging from 0 [not at all] to 3 [very often]).

Once ratings are obtained, scores can be tallied and compared to normative data relative to the referred child's age and gender. If the score for either inattention or hyperactivity/impulsivity exceeds a specific criterion for either parent or teacher ratings, then further evaluation for ADHD may be necessary. The threshold used for screening decisions should be set at a level where NPP is high but that allows for some degree of false-positive identifications. As described previously, Power, Andrews, and colleagues (1998) found the 80th percentile to be the optimal criterion for school-based screening using the ADHD Rating Scale IV. Similar results were found for cutoff scores using a clinic-based sample (Power, Doherty, et al., 1998). Thus, those children whose scores exceed the 80th percentile relative to peers of the same age and gender should receive further evaluation for possible ADHD. Those children whose scores are under the 80th percentile should be evaluated for other possible disorders as ADHD does not appear to be a likely diagnosis.

As an alternative to the norm-referenced approach, ratings could be interpreted regarding the number of ADHD symptoms that are exhibited to a clinically significant degree. Any symptom items reported to occur "often" or "very often" are counted as present, while symptom items receiving endorsements of "not at all" or "sometimes" are counted as absent. If either the parent or teacher reports a symptom as present, then it is counted as present. The number of symptoms present in each category (inattention and hyperactivity/impulsivity) can be tallied and compared to *DSM-IV* criteria. In this fashion, if a child or adolescent is reported to exhibit at least six symptoms of either inattention or hyperactivity/impulsivity, then further evaluation of ADHD is necessary. Given the goal of being inclusive at this stage of the evaluation process, it is desirable to set a more liberal threshold for number of present symptoms in order to continue the evaluation of ADHD. For example, DuPaul and Stoner (2003) suggested that further evaluation should be conducted if at least four symptoms are reported for either inattention or hyperactivity/impulsivity.

A second screening method is to interview either the parent or teacher regarding symptomatic criteria for ADHD. The *DSM-IV* criteria could be reviewed with respondents indicating the degree to which each of the 18 symptoms is exhibited frequently (often or very often). If both the teacher and parent are interviewed and either one reports a symptom as present, it is counted as such. As was the case for behavior ratings, the total number of symptoms reported in each category can be tallied and a decision can be made to conduct further assessment if a given symptom threshold (at least four in either category) is met.

Screening for Comorbid Disorders

Children and adolescents with ADHD are likely to have at least one comorbid behavior or learning disorder as ADHD rarely occurs alone, at least in clinic-referred samples (Barkley, 2006). Thus, a comprehensive evaluation of ADHD should include procedures to screen for comorbid disorders (Anastopoulos & Shelton, 2001; Barkley, 2006). In fact, the AAP (in press) clinical practice guideline for diagnosis, evaluation, and treatment of ADHD recommends that "clinicians should include assessment for other conditions that might coexist with ADHD including emotional or behavioral (e.g., anxiety, depressive, oppositional defiant, and conduct disorders), developmental (e.g., learning and language disorders), and physical (e.g., tics, sleep apnea) conditions." For adolescents, symptoms and signs of substance abuse should also be assessed.

Screening measures for emotional and behavioral disorders should include broad-band and narrow-band rating scales completed by parents, teachers, and children. Broad-band measures are those that include many items canvassing a wide range of possible behavioral or emotional difficulties across both internalizing (e.g., anxiety, depression) and externalizing (e.g., conduct, oppositional) dimensions (Mash & Terdal, 1997). For example, parents and teachers could complete the Child Behavior Checklist (Achenbach, 1997a) or Behavior Assessment System for Children II (Reynolds & Kamphaus, 1998). Each of these rating scales includes two broad-band dimensions (internalizing and externalizing) as well as multiple narrow-band dimensions (e.g., attention problems, conduct problems, anxiety). In similar fashion, referred children or adolescents could complete the Youth Self-Report (Achenbach, 1997b) or Behavior Assessment System for Children II Self-Report (Reynolds & Kamphaus, 1998). Elevations beyond a specific threshold (e.g., 93rd percentile for child's age and gender) on subscales beyond those related to ADHD would indicate that further assessment of a comorbid condition is necessary. Given that the screening process should err on the side of caution (i.e., emphasize sensitivity over specificity), further assessment of comorbidity should occur if the respondent's ratings are elevated on a non-ADHD dimension. For example, if ratings from a child's teacher were beyond the 93rd percentile on a depression subscale, then further evaluation of possible depressive symptomatology would ensue.

One way to further assess for possible comorbid emotion or behavior disorders is to ask respondents to complete a narrow-band rating scale specific to the condition of interest (Anastopoulos & Shelton, 2001). Narrow-band measures tend to be relatively brief with items focused on symptomatic behaviors specific to one or two disorders. Examples of narrow-band measures focused on internalizing symptomatology include the Children's Depression Inventory (Kovacs, 1992), Multidimensional Anxiety Scale for Children (March, Parker, Sullivan, Stallings, & Conners, 1997), Reynolds Child Depression Scale (Reynolds, 1989), and Reynolds Adolescent Depression Scale (Reynolds, 2002). Most narrow-band internalizing rating scales are self-reported measures because children themselves are often in the best position to "observe" symptoms of anxiety and depression. An example of a narrow-band measure focused on externalizing symptoms is the Eyberg Child Behavior Inventory (Eyberg & Pincus, 1999). Narrow-band measures of externalizing behaviors are almost exclusively completed by parents and teachers because children with ADHD tend to be poor reporters of externalizing symptomatology (Barkley, 2006). A clinically significant elevation (e.g., score at or beyond the 93rd percentile) on a narrow-band rating scale typically leads to a more comprehensive evaluation of a possible comorbid disorder.

Screening for a possible learning or language disorder involves several procedures. First, the classroom teacher(s) should be interviewed briefly regarding possible student difficulties with reading, math, and other academic subject areas. Specific information regarding where the student is placed in the curriculum (i.e., grade level), how the student is functioning in relation to classmates, as well as strengths and weaknesses in a given subject matter should be discussed (for more details regarding teacher interview, see Shapiro, 1996). Second, archival data regarding student academic functioning should be examined. For example, recent written assignments and tests could be reviewed. Third, teachers could be asked to complete a brief rating of academic skills such as the Academic Performance Rating Scale (DuPaul, Rapport, & Perriello, 1991) or Academic Competence Evaluation Scale (DiPerna & Elliott, 2000). Finally, a brief direct assessment of student reading and/or math could be conducted using curriculum-based measurement (CBM; Shinn, 1998). CBM probes are relatively brief (e.g., 2–5 minutes) and can help determine a student's status relative to grade-level curriculum.

The combination of these measures can indicate whether more comprehensive assessment of a learning disability is necessary. Evaluation of comorbid learning disability is especially indicated when screening measures indicate consistent performance below grade level and relative to classmates despite teacher modifications in instruction and/or other strategies to address academic deficits.

Roles and Responsibilities of School Personnel and Health Care Providers

School personnel and primary health care providers serve critically important roles in screening for ADHD. These practitioners are typically the first professionals to recognize possible ADHD symptoms and identify those children and adolescents requiring comprehensive evaluation. The chief roles and responsibilities include 1) devising a psychometrically sound, feasible screening process; 2) implementing the screening process when appropriate; 3) making accurate screening decisions; 4) ensuring comprehensive evaluation for children who screen positive; and 5) monitoring the outcome of the evaluation process.

The first responsibility of school and health care professionals is to create an effective screening process. Screening components and processes will vary as a function of the screening, as discussed previously. We have provided guidelines for how screening should be carried out across settings, but there are also many local decisions that need to be reached prior to initiating the screening process. For example, the specific screening measure(s) must be selected, individuals who will facilitate the process should be designated, and appropriate timelines/expectations need to be set. In schools, there are several professionals who could facilitate this process, including the school psychologist, special educator, or school nurse. In primary health care settings, a nurse or office staff member can oversee the screening; in some cases, the primary care physician would serve in this role. The chief point is that all of these decisions should be made proactively so that an efficient, feasible protocol is followed on a consistent basis.

Once a screening protocol is in place, then designated professionals should ensure that this process is followed whenever appropriate. For example, the school psychologist should schedule universal screening at the beginning of each school year and facilitate completion of prescribed activities. Proper implementation will require setting concrete timelines for completion of screening as well as making it clear who will be responsible for administering and collecting screening data. Any problems that arise with implementation should be noted for discussion and possible modification of procedures for future iterations of the screening protocol.

The third responsibility for school and health care professionals is to make accurate decisions based on screening data. Accuracy is enhanced when administration is monitored for adherence with standardized instructions and procedures. Furthermore, scoring accuracy on rating scales or interviews should be checked on at least a random basis (if not for every screening protocol). Finally, scores must be compared with relevant cutpoints to determine whether children require further evaluation. Whenever possible, cutpoints should be based on normative data that are appropriate for a child's age, gender, and ethnicity.

Children and adolescents who screen positive for ADHD should be referred for a comprehensive evaluation. As described in Chapter 4, this evaluation should include multiple methods and respondents. Furthermore, the evaluation must not only focus on ADHD symptoms but also explore other possible reasons (e.g., other disorders) for the child's difficulties. If the evaluation is not conducted in the screening setting (i.e., school or primary health care clinic), then families must be referred to a professional who has established expertise in evaluating ADHD and related disorders. In such cases, school and health care professionals should check with the family to make sure that the evaluation actually takes place and that results are available in a timely fashion.

The final responsibility is to monitor the outcome of the evaluation process with specific emphasis on ensuring that children receive appropriate treatment based on assessment results. The designated school or health care professional overseeing the screening process should review evaluation reports and work with families to obtain recommended interventions. In the school setting, it may require consulting with classroom teachers to devise, implement, and evaluate classroom strategies. In the health care clinic, it may involve prescribing appropriate medication and/or providing parent training.

Communication Among Families, Schools, and Health Care Providers

For ADHD screening to be effective, communication among families, schools, and health care providers is critically important. Individuals across all three settings (i.e., home, school, health care clinic) will be involved, especially in cases where children screen positive for ADHD. The three elements of communication that are most important include clarity, respect, and timeliness.

First, all communication regarding the content and process of screening should be as clear as possible. When working with parents, practitioners should explain the reason for screening and expectations for parental input in everyday, jargon-free language. It is important to review the possible steps in the screening process, especially in cases where a positive screen might be obtained. In addition, the parent's questions should be solicited and answered to ensure complete understanding. A similar process should be followed when soliciting teacher input. Parents and teachers should be informed that a positive screen does not mean that a child will be diagnosed with ADHD, but rather this indicates that further assessment is necessary. When educational and health care personnel communicate during the screening process, each should avoid using their specific professional jargon so that mutual understanding is enhanced.

It is critical that individuals involved in the screening process strive to treat each other with as much respect as possible. Each participant brings expertise to the process as parents are most knowledgeable of their children's home behavior and history, teachers are familiar with classroom norms and expectations as well as children's day-to-day performance, other school professionals (e.g., school psychologists) have necessary experience with assessment methods, and health care staff are experts with respect to children's health and development. The fact that some parents may exhibit ADHD symptoms or other difficulties themselves does not obviate the need to be respectful when soliciting and reviewing their input. Cultural, linguistic, and ethnic differences need to be accounted for as part of this process. For example, if English is not the primary language spoken in the home, then screening measures should be administered in the parents' primary language. In this case, family culture is respected and the probability of obtaining accurate parent input is increased.

Communication should be made in as timely a manner as possible. The screening process involves several steps, and it is important these are completed within a reasonable time period so that treatment can be provided when necessary. Thus, parents should be contacted to provide informed consent and screening input as soon as possible. Parents and teachers should be provided with reasonable but timely deadlines (e.g., 1 week) to complete screening measures. Given that most measures do not require more than 10 minutes to complete, this is not an onerous request. Parent and teacher questions should be answered as quickly as possible so as to ensure ongoing collaboration. Finally, screening results should be provided to all participants within a reasonable time period. Again, given that scoring and interpretation of most measures only requires a few minutes, it should not take more than a day or two to provide participants with results and discussion of next steps, when necessary. In general, the more efficiently each step is followed and communicated, the greater the probability that participants will work collaboratively on any subsequent endeavors (i.e., comprehensive evaluation, treatment planning, treatment implementation).

Conclusions

Screening for ADHD is important because earlier identification and treatment may increase chances for success and help to prevent problematic outcomes. Although the symptoms of this disorder are overt, noticeable, and likely to lead to referral, epidemiological data indicate that a significant proportion of the ADHD population goes unrecognized and untreated. There are at least three situations for which screening should take place: universal screening for ADHD in early elementary school, individual screening for ADHD when children are referred for learning and behavior problems, and individual screening for comorbid disorders when children and adolescents are identified with ADHD. Brief, psychometrically sound screening measures include parent and teacher ratings of ADHD symptoms. Diagnostic interview data from parents and/or teachers can also aid in the screening process. It is important that a clear, feasible screening process is designed and implemented in schools and primary health care practices as these are the settings where "first responders" to ADHD are located. Screening decisions should be empirically based and linked to comprehensive assessment when positive screens are obtained. Ultimately, the effectiveness of screening is dependent on providing appropriate treatment to those children and adolescents who require such services.

References

Achenbach, T.M. (1997a). *Manual for the Child Behavior Checklist and Revised Child Behavior Profile*. Burlington: University of Vermont, Department of Psychiatry.

Achenbach, T.M. (1997b). *Manual for the Youth Self-Report*. Burlington: University of Vermont, Department of Psychiatry.

American Academy of Pediatrics. (in press). Clinical practice guideline: Diagnosis, evaluation, and treatment of the child and adolescent with attention-deficit/hyperactivity disorder. *Pediatrics*.

American Psychiatric Association. (1994). *Diagnostic and statistical manual of mental disorders* (4th ed.). Washington, DC: Author.

Anastopoulos, A.D., & Shelton, T.L. (2001). *Assessing attention-deficit/hyperactivity disorder*. New York: Kluwer Academic/Plenum.

Barkley, R.A. (Ed.). (2006). *Attention-deficit/hyperactivity disorder: A handbook for diagnosis and treatment* (3rd ed.). New York: Guilford Press.

Boyce, W.T., Essex, M.J., Goldstein, L.H., Armstrong, J.M., Kraemer, H.C., & Kupfer, D.J. (2002). The confluence of mental, physical, social, and academic difficulties of middle childhood: I. Exploring the "headwaters" of early life morbidities. *Journal of the American Academy of Child and Adolescent Psychiatry, 41*, 580–587.

Bussing, R., Fernandez, M., Harwood, M., Hou, W., Garvan, C.W., Eyberg, S.M., et al. (2008). Parent and teacher SNAP-IV ratings of attention deficit hyperactivity disorder symptoms: Psychometric properties and normative ratings from a school district sample. *Assessment, 15,* 317–328.

Conners, C.K. (1969). A teacher rating scale for use in drug studies with children. *American Journal of Psychiatry, 126*, 884–888.

DiPerna, J.C., & Elliott, S.N. (2000). *Academic Competence Evaluation Scale.* San Antonio, TX: Psychological Corporation.

DuPaul, G.J., Power, T.J., Anastopoulos, A.D., & Reid, R. (1998). *ADHD Rating Scale-IV: Checklists, norms, and clinical interpretation.* New York: Guilford Press.

DuPaul, G.J., Rapport, M.D., & Perriello, L.M. (1991). Teacher ratings of academic skills: The development of the Academic Performance Rating Scale. *School Psychology Review, 20*, 284–300.

DuPaul, G.J., & Stoner, G. (2003). *ADHD in the schools: Assessment and intervention strategies* (2nd ed.). New York: Guilford Press.

Epstein, J.N., March, J.S., Conners, C.K., & Jackson, D.L. (1998). Racial differences on the Conners Teacher Rating Scale. *Journal of Abnormal Child Psychology, 26*, 109–118.

Essex, M.J., Kraemer, H.C., Slattery, M.J., Burk, L.R., Boyce, W.T., Woodward, H.R., et al. (2009). Screening for childhood mental health problems: Outcomes and early identification. *Journal of Child Psychology and Psychiatry, 50*, 562–570.

Eyberg, S.M., & Pincus, D. (1999). *Eyberg Child Behavior Inventory and Sutter-Eyberg Student Behavior Inventory: Professional manual.* Odessa, FL: Psychological Assessment Resources.

Froehlich, T.E., Lanphear, B.P., Epstein, J.N., Barbaresi, W.J., Katusic, S.K., & Kahn, R.S. (2007). Prevalence, recognition, and treatment of attention-deficit/hyperactivity disorder in a national sample in US children. *Archives of Pediatric and Adolescent Medicine, 161*, 857–864.

Gadow, K.D., & Sprafkin, J. (1997). *ADHD Symptom Checklist 4 manual.* Stony Brook, NY: Checkmate Plus.

Gardner, W., Lucas, A., Kolko, D.J., & Campo, J.V. (2007). Comparison of the PSC-17 and alternative mental health screens in an at-risk primary care sample. *Journal of the American Academy of Child and Adolescent Psychiatry, 46*, 611–618.

Goodman, R. (2001). Psychometric properties of the Strengths and Difficulties Questionnaire (SDQ). *Journal of the American Academy of Child and Adolescent Psychiatry, 40*, 1337–1345.

Jellinek, M.S., Murphy, J.M., Little, M., Pagano, M.E., Comer, D.M., & Kelleher, K.J. (1999). Use of the Pediatric Symptom Checklist to screen for psychosocial problems in pediatric primary care: A national feasibility study. *Archives in Pediatrics and Adolescent Medicine, 153*, 254–260.

Kovacs, M. (1992). *Children's Depression Inventory (CDI) manual.* Tonowanda, NY: Multi-Health Systems.

March, J.S., Parker, J.D., Sullivan, K., Stallings, P., & Conners, C.K. (1997). The Multidimensional Anxiety Scale for Children (MASC): Factor structure, reliability, and validity. *Journal of the American Academy of Child and Adolescent Psychiatry, 36*, 554–565.

Mash, E.J., & Terdal, L.G. (Eds.). (1997). *Assessment of childhood disorders* (3rd ed.). New York: Guilford Press.

Pastor, P.N., & Reuben, C.A. (2008). Diagnosed attention deficit hyperactivity disorder and learning disability: United States, 2004–2006. *Vital Health Statistics, 10*, 1–14.

Pelham, W.E., Gnagy, E.M., Greenslade, K.E., & Milich, R. (1992). Teacher ratings of DSM-III-R symptoms for the disruptive behavior disorders. *Journal of the American Academy of Child & Adolescent Psychiatry, 31*, 210–218.

Polanczyk, G., Silva de Lima, M., Horta, B.L., Biederman, J., & Rohde, L.A. (2007). The worldwide prevalence of ADHD: A systematic review and metaregression analysis. *American Journal of Psychiatry, 164*, 942–948.

Power, T.J., Andrews, T.J., Eiraldi, R.B., Doherty, B.J., Ikeda, M.J., DuPaul, G.J., et al. (1998). Evaluating attention deficit hyperactivity disorder using multiple informants: The incremental utility of combining teacher with parent reports. *Psychological Assessment, 10*, 250–260.

Power, T.J., Doherty, B.J., Panichelli-Mindel, S.M., Karustis, J.L., Eiraldi, R.B., Anastopoulos, A.D., et al. (1998). The predictive validity of parent and teacher reports of ADHD symptoms. *Journal of Psychopathology and Behavioral Assessment, 20*, 57–81.

Reid, R., DuPaul, G.J., Power, T.J., Anastopoulos, A.D., & Riccio, C. (1998). Assessing culturally different students for attention deficit hyperactivity disorder using behavior rating scales. *Journal of Abnormal Child Psychology, 26*, 187–198.

Reynolds, C.R., & Kamphaus, R.W. (1998). *Behavior Assessment System for Children Manual* (2nd ed.). Circle Pines, MN: American Guidance Service.

Reynolds, W.M. (1989). *Reynolds Child Depression Scale: Professional manual.* Odessa, FL: Psychological Assessment Resources.

Reynolds, W.M. (2002). *Reynolds Adolescent Depression Scale: Professional manual* (2nd ed.). Odessa, FL: Psychological Assessment Resources.

Satin, M.S., Winsberg, B.G., Monetti, C.H., Sverd, J., & Foss, D.A. (1985). A general population screen for attention deficit disorder with hyperactivity. *Journal of the American Academy of Child and Adolescent Psychiatry, 24*, 756–764.

Shapiro, E.S. (1996). *Academic skills problems: Direct assessment and intervention (2nd ed.).* New York: Guilford Press.

Shinn, M.R. (Ed.). (1998). *Advanced applications of curriculum-based measurement.* New York: Guilford.

Swanson, J.M. (1992). *School-based assessments and interventions for ADD students.* Irvine, CA: KC Publications.

Walker, H.M., & Severson, H. (1988). *Systematic screening for behavior disorders assessment system.* Longmont, CO: Sopris West.

Wolraich, M.L., Feurer, I.D., Hannah, J.N., Baumgartel, A., & Pinnock, T.Y. (1998). Obtaining systematic teacher reports of disruptive behavior disorders utilizing DSM-IV. *Journal of Abnormal Child Psychology, 26*, 141–152.

Wolraich, M.L., Lambert, W., Doffing, M.A., Bickman, L., Simmons, T., & Worley, K. (2003). Psychometric properties of the Vanderbilt ADHD diagnostic parent rating scale in a referred population. *Journal of Pediatric Psychology, 28*, 559–568.

CHAPTER 4

Diagnosis

The diagnostic process for evaluating children for attention-deficit/hyperactivity disorder (ADHD) generally occurs in one or two of three settings. The diagnosis leading to treatment with medication or with home-based behavioral interventions generally occurs in primary care or mental health settings, while evaluations to obtain educational services (e.g., academic and behavioral interventions) occur in school settings. Children with less severe ADHD who have no or less severe co-occurring conditions can be diagnosed by their primary care clinician. However, children with more severe ADHD—particularly those with complicating co-occurring conditions—require evaluation from a mental health clinician. School evaluations primarily focus on a child's educational needs, particularly the identification of conditions that impair a child's ability to learn in the classroom. Ideally, all evaluations are accomplished with an interdisciplinary team that includes multiple clinicians covering health, mental health, and educational aspects. However, such evaluation teams have become uncommon because of the increased difficulty in finding programs that can support such evaluations and their expense. Because most evaluations are now completed by individual clinicians, communication between professionals and parents is critically important (see Chapter 8).

The diagnostic evaluation starts with making use of the information collected in the screening process discussed in Chapter 3. It requires identifying the presence of specific behaviors that impair a child's functioning. Even though ADHD is a neurobiologic condition with strong evidence for a substantial genetic contribution and with differences in brain structure and function, there are no laboratory tests or neuroimaging indices available to help establish a definitive and reliable diagnosis. In addition, because the symptoms that are assessed are behaviors that sometimes occur in children who do not have ADHD, it is important to determine the frequency of the behaviors in different settings compared to the expected frequencies in children who do not have ADHD. Because ADHD-related behaviors are very susceptible to effects of the environmental context, it is not reliable to solely depend on short episodes of observations, even though such observations can be obtained with more precision.

Although the current diagnostic system, the *Diagnostic and Statistical Manual of Mental Disorders, Fourth Edition, Text Revision* (*DSM-IV-TR*; American Psychiatric Association [APA], 2000), does not specify how to collect assessment data, the best results are obtained by querying those individuals who have the most extensive contact with the child, usually parents and teachers. The American Academy of Pediatrics (AAP, 2000) in its guideline for diagnosing ADHD has specifically recommended to obtain information from both the teacher and parent whenever possible for determining the diagnosis. It is therefore essential that clinicians and teachers communicate during the diagnostic process (see Chapter 8).

This chapter first describes the criteria required in establishing a diagnosis of ADHD. It then discusses the difficulties and challenges in making the diagnosis. Finally, it presents the characteristics of other behavioral and cognitive conditions that can frequently co-occur in children who have the diagnosis of ADHD.

Specific Criteria

To make the diagnosis of ADHD, the clinician needs to determine the presence of behaviors as outlined by the most recent changes in criteria in the *DSM-IV-TR*. These criteria include two dimensions: inattention and hyperactivity-impulsivity. Behaviors specific to each dimension are characterized in Table 4.1. The clinician needs to determine how many of the core symptoms are occurring, as well as the extent to which these symptoms cause impairment in multiple settings, particularly home and school.

An individual's symptoms are clinically significant if the individual displays six of the nine behaviors in each dimension at a frequency that is inappropriate for his or her developmental level and gender. Given

Table 4.1. Core symptoms of attention-deficit/hyperactivity disorder (ADHD)

Inattention dimension	Hyperactivity-impulsivity dimension	
	Hyperactivity	*Impulsivity*
Careless mistakes	Fidgeting	Blurting answers before
Difficulty sustaining attention	Unable to stay seated	questions completed
Seems not to listen	Moving excessively (restless)	Difficulty awaiting turn
Fails to finish tasks		Interrupting/intruding upon others
Difficulty organizing	Difficulty engaging in leisure activities quietly	
Avoids tasks requiring sustained attention	"On the go"	
Loses things	Talking excessively	
Easily distracted		
Forgetful		

the ubiquitous finding of gender differences in ADHD symptom frequency, with boys displaying these behaviors more frequently than girls (e.g., DuPaul et al., 1997), the appropriateness of each symptom dimension should also be considered relative to established gender norms (e.g., for behavior rating scales completed by parents and teachers).

Sources of Information

The diagnosis of ADHD remains dependent on obtaining information about a patient's behavior from those who most frequently observe the behavior. As noted previously, because teachers observe children for up to 6 hours per day in comparison to a group of same-age peers and in situations that require children to pay attention and control their activity level and impulsivity, they are important reporters. When possible, it is also helpful to obtain information from other observers, such as coaches, scout leaders, and grandparents. Direct observations of a child's behavior in the classroom can provide some of the most objective information if it is available, but as noted previously, it can only capture a limited amount of observed time because it is labor intensive. Limited observations frequently may not reflect the overall pattern of behavior because the child's activities tend to be very influenced by the environmental situation. This issue probably explains why observations in clinical situations such as a doctor's office may not provide an accurate picture of a child's overall behaviors (Sleator, Neumann, & Sprague,

1974). In addition, the clinical evaluation is frequently a novel situation for a child, so the child's behavior may not be typical of behavior in familiar surroundings.

Unfortunately, children are not reliable reporters of their own behaviors, which they tend to underreport (Hoza, Pelham, Dobbs, Owens, & Pillow, 2002). This finding is true both in younger children and in adolescents (Smith, Pelham, Gnagy, Molina, & Evans, 2000). With adolescents, it is more difficult to obtain accurate information from other sources because parents have fewer opportunities to observe their teenagers. By middle school and high school, students frequently have multiple teachers who only observe them for limited times each day. When possible, it is still best to have both teacher and parent input. Two or three teachers of the most critical academic subjects (i.e., math, English, science, social studies) should complete ratings either independently or as a team. It is also important to determine how well adolescents are able to monitor their own behavior.

There may be disagreement regarding symptom frequency and severity, as well as degree of impairment between parents and teachers (Mitsis, McKay, Schulz, Newcorn, & Halperin, 2000). To a great degree, the disagreement probably relates to the different situations in which teachers and parents observe their children. When there is significant disagreement, it is helpful to try to determine which individuals are providing the most accurate perceptions. Biases can be present with the parent, the teacher, or both. Some suggestions for how to clarify differences in parent and teacher reports are presented in Table 4.2.

Table 4.2.   Evaluating reporter disagreement

Review the behaviors (at least with the parent) to ensure that the reporter is accurately observing the specific behaviors.

Obtain information from additional sources, including previous teachers, current ancillary teachers, aides, coaches, scout or organizational leaders, religious teachers, the other parent or stepparent, and other relatives.

Get a report of the child's behavior during psychoeducational assessments or interventions.

Determine if the parents or teachers are strongly opinionated either for or against stimulant medication.

If the child is an only child or the oldest in the family, determine whether the parents have appropriate expectations for behavior based on the child's developmental level.

Determine the experience level of the teacher. Teachers with more years in the classroom may rate behavioral symptoms in a more appropriate developmental context than those with lesser experience.

Other Criteria

In addition to the core symptoms, patients with ADHD must meet the criteria presented in Table 4.3. ADHD is classified as one of three subtypes depending on what core symptoms are present:

- *Predominantly inattentive type:* children who meet the criteria on the inattentive dimension (six or more of nine inattentive core symptoms)

- *Predominantly hyperactive/impulsive type:* children who meet the criteria on the hyperactivity/impulsivity dimension (six or more of nine hyperactive/impulsive core symptoms)

- *Combined type:* children who meet six of the nine criteria on both dimensions

The age requirement of 7 years is included to reflect a biologic basis for the condition starting in childhood. The age is not empirically derived. Some children with the inattentive subtype may not present (or show symptoms) until an older age, when they have a greater need to be able to concentrate. In addition, with some children, the symptoms may have been present at a younger age but were not felt to be abnormal or the manifestations went undiagnosed. Thus, some researchers have argued for the use of childhood onset (i.e., prior to 18 years old) for symptoms rather than age 7 (Barkley & Biederman, 1997). The duration requirement of 6 months reflects the chronic nature of the condition. The patterns of behaviors have some variations but are generally consistent, unlike depression, for which symptoms are more likely to be episodic. The most important aspect of the diagnosis is the concept that the core symptoms impair the child's ability to function. There are individuals who have many of the core symptoms, but because of their strengths (e.g., above-average intelligence), they are able to compensate well enough to prevent the symptoms from causing significant dysfunction. Assessment of function is discussed in more detail in Chapter 5.

Table 4.3.   Other criteria for attention-deficit/hyperactivity disorder (ADHD)

Some hyperactive/impulsive or inattentive symptoms that caused impairment present before 7 years of age

Symptoms have persisted for at least 6 months

Some impairment from the symptoms is present in two or more settings (e.g., home, school, work)

Evidence for clinically significant impairment in social, academic, or occupational functioning due to the behaviors

Based on *DSM-IV-TR*, a diagnosis of ADHD should not be made if a diagnosis of pervasive developmental disorder (an autism spectrum disorder) and childhood schizophrenia is warranted. Particularly, children with autism spectrum disorder may display a number of core ADHD symptoms. Although they are less likely to have a beneficial response to treatment for ADHD, some will show improvement with medications used to treat children with ADHD (Handen, Johnson, & Lubetsky, 2000; Jahromi et al., 2009). Other behavioral conditions, such as mood and anxiety disorders and learning disabilities, may be the underlying cause of ADHD-like behaviors, but these conditions can also co-occur with ADHD and occur more frequently in children with ADHD than they do in the general population.

Challenges in Establishing the Diagnosis

Making the diagnosis of ADHD can be challenging. The current diagnostic criteria for ADHD are less than perfect even if they are the current state of the art. First, the *DSM* system does not include a developmental perspective; that is, it does not describe different manifestations of the disorder for each age or developmental level of the child. The diagnostic criteria were derived primarily from research in children 6–13 years of age. In preschool-age children (4–6 years of age), the *DSM-IV-TR* diagnostic criteria appear to be appropriate (Egger, Kondo, & Angold, 2006). However, when evaluating adolescents, the clinician frequently is trying to base a diagnosis on retrospective recall of the patient to determine if impairing symptoms were present in childhood. The 18 core symptoms are derived from field trials in children ranging from 4 to 17 years of age. However, some of the behaviors are not appropriately worded for adolescents, such as *runs or climbs excessively* (Lahey et al., 1994).

The symptomatic behaviors are also contextually dependent. The greater the ratio of adults to children, the stronger the interest level of the activity, or the greater the structure in the environment, the easier it is for children to control their behaviors. There are also no specific guidelines for an observer, such as a parent or teacher, to precisely decide that a behavior is occurring inappropriately often. Therefore, the reporting of symptoms is to some extent subjective, and the finding mentioned earlier about discrepancies between parent and teacher reports are not surprising. Generally, teacher reports have correlated well with direct observations of children in the classroom (Danforth & DuPaul, 1996). The teacher's reports in elementary school are likely to be more accurate than those of teachers in middle or high school because they are likely to observe children for a much longer portion of the day.

An additional diagnostic challenge is that the behaviors are not an all-or-none phenomenon. Some of the symptoms may represent typical child behavior depending on the age and gender of the child and the circumstance. Children with difficult temperaments may exhibit behaviors that create problems, but their symptoms—and more importantly their degree of dysfunction—are not severe enough to warrant a diagnosis of ADHD. These difficulties have been referred to as *subsyndromal* and have been defined as inattentive and hyperactive/impulsive problems (Wolraich, Felice, & Drotar, 1996).

Many of the symptomatic behaviors will decrease with age, so in adolescents it is less common to see the hyperactive symptoms; impulsivity also tends to decrease, although fidgeting and squirming, difficulty engaging in quiet leisure activities, and interrupting other people can persist (Barkley, Anastopoulos, Guevremont, & Fletcher, 1991). Adolescents may also experience hyperactivity through feelings of internal restlessness (Weyandt et al., 2003). The symptoms of inattention and difficulties with executive function, while also diminishing with age, are likely to continue into adulthood, although some children are successful at accommodating for these deficits as they mature. Inattention symptoms that frequently persist are paying close attention to details, sustaining attention with tasks, and following through with instructions (Barkley et al., 1991).

It is important to obtain enough information to make a diagnosis based on *DSM-IV-TR* criteria. Using rating scales that base their behavioral symptoms on *DSM* criteria can help to shorten the time required to obtain the information (see Chapter 3). Rating scales also provide useful information for making a diagnosis but only provide some of the information and should not be used as exclusive diagnostic tools without at least reviewing the core behaviors in direct interview with the parents. These scales are particularly helpful in obtaining information from teachers, where other forms of contact may be difficult. As noted in Chapter 3, there are several scales available, including the Vanderbilt Parent and Teacher ADHD Rating Scale (Wolraich et al., 1998; see http://devbehavpeds.ouhsc.edu/rokplay.asp), the ADHD Rating Scale IV (DuPaul, Power, Anastopoulos, & Reid, 1998), the Swanson, Nolan, and Pelham (SNAP) IV (Swanson, Nolan, & Pelham, 1981; see http://www.adhd.net/) and the Revised Conners Teacher and Parent Rating Scales (Conners, 1969).

Other laboratory tests or imaging studies have not been found to be useful in making the specific diagnosis, although they may be useful if some co-occurring condition is considered. For example, for exposure to lead, it is important to screen children with ADHD as you would other children if they live in an at-risk area. Thyroid abnormalities are not likely to be present without other thyroid symptoms. The standard electroencephalograms (EEG) are helpful in diagnosing seizures if the information obtained from parents suggests symptoms that could be seizures. Although there is an increased incidence of nonspecific EEG changes in children with ADHD, they have little diagnostic utility at this time (Chabot, di Michele, & Prichep, 2005). Computerized EEG assessments are used for research purposes, but they have not been found to contribute to making a diagnosis (AAP, 2000).

Many children with ADHD will also have poor coordination in their fine and/or gross motor skills (Fliers et al., 2008). These findings used to be called "soft neurological signs" because part of the manifestation was the retention of signs (e.g., not distinguishing left from right) beyond the expected age when they should disappear. Deficits in coordination have been referred to as *developmental coordination disorder* or *motor dysfunction.* These deficits are important to identify because they can impair social functions, such as the child's performance in athletic activities, and academic performance in writing.

An assessment of academic and social functioning is a required component in establishing the ADHD diagnosis (see Chapter 5). Some behavior rating scales that assess ADHD symptoms also include questions relating to function. The second section of the Vanderbilt Parent and Teacher ADHD Rating Scale provides information about functioning. The SNAP is usually administered with the Swanson, Kotkin, Agler, M-Flynn, and Pelham Scale (SKAMP) (Murray et al., 2009), which assesses function. The SKAMP is available from the same source as the SNAP. In addition, both the parent and child should be asked about how well the child is doing in the domains of peer and family relations and academic, community (organized activities), and leisure functioning.

Diagnosis of Comorbid Conditions

Because co-occurring behavioral and physical conditions are common in patients with ADHD, it is very important that clinician's diagnostic process not only determine that a patient has the diagnosis of ADHD and does not have another diagnosis, but also if other common co-occurring conditions are present. *Comorbidity* is the term that the *DSM-IV-TR* uses to refer to disorders that are present at the same time as the diagnosis of ADHD and are not the cause of the ADHD symptoms. The majority of individuals with ADHD will have at least one other comorbid condition (Barkley, 2006).

The comorbid conditions can be categorized into four groups: 1) cognitive, 2) behavioral or mental, 3) motoric, and 4) physical disorders. They are discussed in more detail in the following section. These four categories emphasize the importance of an integrated health education process for evaluating children suspected of having ADHD. The health care system is important in assessing the physical disorders, whereas the schools are frequently the best source for assessing the cognitive disorders. Both systems may assess the motoric and behavioral or mental disorders. The cognitive deficits include learning and language disorders. The behavioral or mental disorders are further divided into internalizing and externalizing conditions. The motoric conditions include tic and developmental coordination disorders. In addition, there are some physical conditions that can frequently co-occur, such as unresponsiveness to thyroid hormone.

Learning Disabilities

Learning disabilities are specific cognitive deficits that interfere with some aspects of learning or academic performance such that the individual is not able to achieve up to his or her overall cognitive abilities. The deficits can be in any academic activity (e.g., reading, written expression, mathematics), although the most common disability is in reading. Individuals with learning disabilities in reading (dyslexia) most frequently have weaknesses in their ability to discriminate sounds in words, referred to as phonologic awareness. A language deficit is also frequently associated with reading disability. Learning disabilities can be suspected even before children start school if a child appears delayed in learning letters, numbers, or colors. The previous idea that letter reversal is the major characteristic of a learning disability is not correct because mild continuation of letter reversal or substitute letters occurs in children who do not have learning disabilities. Language deficits frequently are related to the practical use of language referred to as pragmatics and may not be detected with traditional speech and language evaluations. Evaluations by speech clinicians examining how children use language in their day-to-day activities may be needed.

Children suspected of having a learning disability historically have been evaluated with a psychoeducational battery of tests to characterize their cognitive and academic skills. This battery typically includes, at a minimum, a standardized individual general test of intelligence, such as the Wechsler Intelligence Scale for Children, Fourth Edition (Wechsler,

2003), and an individualized standard achievement test, such as the Woodcock-Johnson III Tests of Achievement (Woodcock, McGrew, & Mather, 2000). The assessment for such conditions is what is completed by the school system in considering a child for special education services. More recently, some schools first have tried less intense interventions to further clarify the extent of the problem before employing a formal evaluation. This response to intervention (RTI) approach places an emphasis on identifying effective instructional strategies that can be used in general education classrooms. The assumption of the RTI approach is that those students who do not respond to good instruction, especially when intensified and individualized, may have a learning disability that warrants special education.

For health professionals who are evaluating children for ADHD, an informal screen can include determining children's grades and annual group achievement test results, as well as checking with the parents and teachers to determine if they think children are performing satisfactorily and up to their potential. It is helpful for health and mental health clinicians to know the school system's procedures on assessing children for learning disabilities. Given the demands that some schools face with limited funding, completing assessments in a timely manner may be a challenge. It may take some prodding by the parents to ensure that their child's difficulties are addressed with an RTI approach and/or evaluated in a timely fashion. The clinician can help by providing parents with information about the process and educational requirements. Negotiated procedures between the school system and the health care providers can help to reduce misunderstandings and family conflicts with the systems (see Chapter 8).

Low cognitive abilities that in the past were referred to as "mental retardation" are not a contraindication for diagnosing or treating a child with ADHD (Gadow, 1985). The severity and frequency of possible ADHD symptoms are evaluated relative to others of the same mental age rather than comparing with peers of the same chronological age (Barkley, 2006). Stimulant medications can be beneficial for children with intellectual disabilities and ADHD, although they are not as efficacious in those children with more severe limitations (Aman, Marks, Turbott, Wilsher, & Merry, 1991). The same psychoeducational evaluation used to diagnose learning disabilities will also identify intellectual limitations.

Externalizing Conditions

The next most common group of comorbid behavioral conditions are the externalizing conditions, or disruptive behavior disorders. In addition to ADHD, the other externalizing conditions are oppositional defiant disorder (ODD) and conduct disorder (CD). ODD is a milder manifestation of CD and is frequently the first presentation seen in children who subsequently develop CD. The criteria require at least four of the following defiant and disruptive behaviors that occur often, last greater than half a year, and are greater than would be anticipated by the child's mental abilities:

1. Loses temper

2. Argues with adult

3. Actively defies or refuses to follow rules or comply with requests by adults

4. Is intentionally annoying to people

5. Blames others for his or her mistakes

6. Is touchy or easily annoyed by others

7. Is angry or resentful

8. Is spiteful or vindictive

The symptoms may diminish as the child's ADHD is treated with stimulant medication. However, parents and teachers typically require some training in behavior management to adequately address the child's noncompliant, oppositional behavior.

CD is essentially a more severe manifestation of antisocial behaviors and is characterized by behaviors that violate the rights of others and the norms of society. The behaviors relating to aggression include the following:

- Bullying
- Starting physical fights
- Using weapons to cause physical harm
- Being physically cruel to people
- Being cruel to animals
- Stealing with direct confrontation of the victims
- Forcing an individual into sexual activity.

The behaviors that relate to theft, deceit, or destroying property include the following:

- Breaking into another individual's property (e.g., house, car)
- Often lying to obtain things or avoid obligations
- Stealing without confronting the other individual
- Deliberately setting fire

- Deliberately destroying other individuals' property

Serious violations of rules include the following:

- Often staying out without parent permission starting prior to 13 years of age

- Running away from home more than once and skipping school without permission starting before 13 years of age

Three of any of these behaviors occurring in the past year with at least one in the past 6 months that caused significant impairment are required to make the diagnosis. The child needs to provide a repeated pattern of behaviors that interfere with the basic rights of others or violate age-appropriate societal norms. The disturbances in behavior must cause clinically significant impairment in social, academic, or occupational functioning.

CD is not diagnosed if the individual is older than 18 years of age and meets the criteria for antisocial personality disorder. Children with CD have more significant problems with comorbidity with both ADHD and depression. They are also at greater risk for substance abuse, and 25%–40% will eventually develop antisocial personality disorders. Many children will require intense coordinated services such as multisystem therapy (Shepperd et al., 2009).

Internalizing Conditions

There are two major types of internalizing conditions: mood and anxiety disorders.

Mood Disorders

The mood disorders are primarily characterized by major depressive episodes and manic episodes. Whereas the main source of information for the disruptive behavior disorders are parents and teachers, for internalizing symptoms, children and adolescents are a very important source. The feelings of depression or anxiety may have fewer outward behavior manifestations; therefore, interviews and self-report questionnaires are important in establishing a diagnosis. The behavioral criteria for adults are still generally applicable for children with the exceptions that 1) irritability can be present instead of depressed mood and 2) failure to gain appropriate weight only needs to occur over 1 year's duration for dysthmia (lack of emotion). There are nine behaviors; five or more need to have occurred for at least 2 weeks duration. These symptoms include the following:

1. Depressed or irritable mood

2. Diminished interest or pleasure in almost all activities

3. Significant weight loss or gain when not intentionally dieting or not gaining appropriately for age

4. Problems sleeping or sleeping too much almost every day

5. Slowing down or being overactive almost every day that is noticeable to other people

6. Feeling fatigued nearly every day

7. Feeling worthless or excessively and inappropriately guilty

8. Not being able to concentrate or being indecisive most days

9. Thinking about dying or having suicidal thoughts or actions.

One or more major depressive episodes will occur in a major depressive disorder. However, if the symptoms are more chronic (i.e., lasting at least 2 years) and there are symptoms (two or more) but no major depressive episodes, it is referred to as a dysthymic disorder.

If the major depressive episodes are present between manic episodes, an individual has a bipolar disorder. Sometimes an individual may have manic episodes without depression initially and may appear to have ADHD. A family history of bipolar disorder places an individual at higher risk, so the clinician should have a greater sensitivity to the possibility of bipolar disorder if the individual has a positive family history.

Mania is characterized by episodes of three or more of the following symptoms:

1. Having an inflated self-esteem which is described as "grandiosity"

2. Having a decreased need for sleep

3. Being more talkative than usual with what seems like pressure to keep talking

4. Having a flight of ideas (described by the child as their thoughts are racing)

5. Being distracted

6. Having increased activity to achieve a goal or becoming more agitated

7. Having excessive involvement in pleasurable activities that have a high risk for adverse consequences

The symptoms of bipolar disorder are less clear in children than they are in adolescents and adults (Cummings & Fristad, 2008). However, it is important to consider the possibility of bipolar disorder in children with a strong family history for this condition, as well as children who are unresponsive to ADHD treatments and exhibit excessive anger and oppositional behavior.

Anxiety Disorders

Anxiety disorders may also co-occur with ADHD in about 25%–35% of cases (Barkley, 2006). Anxiety disorders include phobias, panic attacks, posttraumatic stress disorder (PTSD), generalized anxiety disorder, separation anxiety disorder, and obsessive-compulsive disorder (OCD). The presence of a comorbid anxiety disorder may indicate the need for a combined psychosocial-psychopharmacological treatment package because these children are found to be more responsive to combined treatment relative to either approach in isolation (March et al., 2000).

Phobias   Phobias are marked, persistent, and excessive or unreasonable fears of specific types (e.g., spiders, darkness, blood injection injury) or situations or of social situations (social phobias). Exposure to the phobic stimulus causes an immediate anxiety response even though the individual realizes that the response is excessive or unreasonable.

Panic Attacks   Panic attacks are discrete periods of intense fear or discomfort of sudden onset. They reach a peak within 10 minutes and are characterized by autonomic responses including palpitations, tachycardia, sweating, cold or hot flushes, and trembling. The individual may experience shortness of breath, chest pain, abdominal distress, dizziness, and paresthesias (abnormal sensation). The individual may fear losing control or dying or feel unreal.

Posttraumatic Stress Disorder   The diagnosis of PTSD requires the individual to have experienced or witnessed an event that involves actual or threatened serious injury or death. The event needs to be persistently reexperienced by recurrent and distressing recollection and dreams of the event causing intense psychological distress and be triggered by cues that symbolize or resemble the event. The individual will persistently avoid the stimuli associated with the trauma but will have persistent symptoms of increased arousal, such as difficulty sleeping, irritability, difficulty with attention, increased vigilance, and exaggerated startle responses.

Generalized Anxiety Disorder   Generalized anxiety disorder includes overanxious disorder of childhood. It is characterized by a general feeling of anxiety not tied to a specific event. The individual may have muscle tension, easy fatigability, irritability, restlessness, difficulty concentrating, and disturbed sleep.

Separation Anxiety Disorder Separation anxiety disorder is a childhood disorder characterized by excessive anxiety when the child is separated from their home or the person to whom they are attached. The anxiety needs to be beyond what would be expected for the child's developmental level and the disturbance needs to last more than 4 weeks. It also must cause significant distress or impairment of function.

Obsessive-Compulsive Disorder OCD is characterized by persistent and recurring thoughts or impulses that are intrusive and inappropriate and cause excessive anxiety. The individual tries to ignore or suppress the thoughts and realizes that they are created by their own mind or tries to neutralize them with other actions that become compulsions (i.e., repetitive behaviors, such as hand washing, that are repeated rigidly) in an attempt to reduce or prevent the distress. In cases where there has been a sudden onset of OCD symptoms, the clinician should consider the possibility of pediatric autoimmune neuropsychiatric disorders associated with streptococcal infections (Swedo et al., 1998).

Motor Disorders

Three motor conditions are commonly comorbid with ADHD. Two are tic disorders, chronic tic disorder and Tourette syndrome, and one is the motor incoordination or dysfunction called developmental coordination disorder.

Chronic Tic Disorder and Tourette Syndrome

Tics are sudden, rapid, nonrhythmic, recurrent, and stereotyped motor or vocal movements that cause marked distress, such as head movements, eye blinking, shoulder shrugging, grunts, or throat clearing. If they last for at least 4 weeks but less than a year, the individual has a transient tic disorder. If they last for more than 12 months but are all motor or all vocal, they constitute a chronic tic disorder. If both motor and verbal tics are present for more than a year and cause marked distress, the individual has Tourette syndrome. The tics can wax and wane, and individuals can voluntarily control them for short periods of time if they concentrate on the control. The most extreme and debilitating form is when the individual cannot resist blurting out highly inappropriate utterances, such as expletives or racial epithets.

Developmental Coordination Disorder

Developmental coordination disorder is a marked impairment in motor coordination not due to a specific motor disorder such as cerebral palsy. Historically it presents as children who do poorly in athletic activities or in fine motor activities. On neurologic examination, the clinician can see problems in hand supination/pronation, finger-to-nose movements, crossing midline, and right-left identification. In children with severe incoordination, it is helpful to obtain an occupational therapy (OT) evaluation. If the child's handwriting is problematic, the OT evaluation may be provided by the school.

Physical Conditions

Some physical conditions are also associated with ADHD. Most individuals with generalized unresponsiveness to thyroid hormone also have ADHD, and many individuals who experience closed head injuries have behaviors compatible with ADHD. In addition, the effects of alcohol can cause ADHD symptoms as part of fetal alcohol syndrome or with fetal alcohol effects. ADHD symptoms also can be seen in fragile X syndrome. It should be noted that these conditions account for a small minority of children with ADHD.

Broad-based rating scales, such as the Conners Parent and Teacher Rating Scales (Conners, Sitarenios, Parker, & Epstein, 1998), the Child Behavior Checklist (Achenbach & Edelbrock, 1991), and the Behavioral Assessment System for Children Second Edition (Reynolds & Kamphouse, 1992), and specific scales such as the Multidimensional Anxiety Scale for Children (van Gastel & Ferdinand, 2008) and the Children's Depression Inventory (Smucker, Craighead, Craighead, & Green, 1986) can be helpful in identifying possible comorbid conditions.

Conclusion

The evaluation of children suspected of having ADHD requires obtaining information about their behaviors from the people who most extensively observe the behaviors—their parents and teachers. It also requires assessment for commonly co-occurring conditions. The process requires obtaining information from parents and teachers through rating scales and interviews; interviews of children and adolescents to determine if any internalizing conditions, such as anxiety and depression, are present; a history of the psychosocial environment of the children; a family history of possible ADHD and any of the commonly co-occurring conditions; a physical and neurological examination; and a history of the children's school performance and any previous psychoeducational assessments. Determining the diagnosis of ADHD is only possible with an extensive evaluation that includes ruling out other causes and determining if other commonly co-occurring conditions are present. Based on a thorough assessment, it is then possible to develop a comprehensive management plan to address ADHD symptoms and associated functional impairments.

References

Achenbach, T., & Edelbrock, L. (1991). *Manual for the Child Behavior Checklist 4-18 and 1991 Profile*. Burlington, VT: University of Vermont.

Aman, M.G., Marks, R.E., Turbott, S.H., Wilsher, C.P., & Merry, S.N. (1991). Clinical effects of methylphenidate and thioridazine in intellectually subaverage children. *Journal of the American Academy of Child and Adolescent Psychiatry, 30,* 246–256.

American Academy of Pediatrics, Committee on Quality Improvement and Subcommittee on Attention-Deficit/Hyperactivity Disorder. (2000). Clinical practice guideline: Diagnosis and evaluation of the child with attention-deficit/hyperactivity disorder. *Pediatrics, 105,* 1158–1170.

American Psychiatric Association. (1994). *Diagnostic and statistical manual of mental disorders* (4th ed.). Washington, DC: Author.

American Psychiatric Association. (2000). *Diagnostic and statistical manual of mental disorders* (4th ed., text rev.). Washington, DC: Author.

Barkley, R. (2006). *Attention-deficit hyperactivity disorder: A handbook for diagnosis and treatment* (3rd ed.). New York: Guilford Press.

Barkley, R.A., Anastopoulos, A.D., Guevremont, D.C., & Fletcher, K.E. (1991). Adolescents with ADHD: Patterns of behavioral adjustment, academic functioning, and treatment utilization. *Journal of the American Academy of Child and Adolescent Psychiatry, 30,* 752–761.

Barkley, R., & Biederman, J. (1997). Toward a broader definition of the age-of-onset criterion for attention-deficit hyperactivity disorder. *Journal of the American Academy of Child and Adolescent Psychiatry, 36*(9), 1204–1210.

Chabot, R., di Michele, F., & Prichep, L. (2005). The role of quantitative electroencephalography in child and adolescent psychiatric disorders. *Child and Adolescent Psychiatric Clinics of North America, 14,* 21–53.

Conners, C.K. (1969). A teacher rating scale for use in drug studies with children. *American Journal of Psychiatry, 126,* 884–888.

Conners, C.K., Sitarenios, G., Parker, J.D., & Epstein, J.N. (1998). Revision and restandardization of the Conners Teacher Rating Scale (CTRS-R): Factor structure, reliability, and criterion validity. *Journal of Abnormal Child Psychology, 26,* 279–291.

Cummings, C., & Fristad, M.A. (2008). Pediatric bipolar disorder: recognition in primary care. *Current Opinion in Pediatrics, 20,* 560–565.

Danforth, J.S., & DuPaul, G.J. (1996). Interrater reliability of teacher rating scales for children with attention deficit hyperactivity disorder. *Journal of Psychopathology and Behavioral Assessment, 18,* 227–237.

DuPaul, G.J., Power, T.J., Anastopoulos, A.D., & Reid, R. (1998). *ADHD Rating Scale IV: Checklists, norms, and clinical interpretation.* New York: Guilford Press.

DuPaul, G.J., Power, T.J., Anastopoulos, A.D., Reid, R., McGoey, K.E., & Ikeda, M.J. (1997). Teacher ratings of attention deficit hyperactivity disorder symptoms: Factor structure and normative data. *Psychological Assessment, 9,* 436–444.

Egger, H.L., Kondo, D., & Angold, A. (2006). The epidemiology and diagnostic issues in preschool attention-deficit/hyperactivity disorder. *Infants and Young Children, 19,* 109–122.

Fliers, E., Rommelse, N., Vermeulen, S.H., Altink, M., Buschgens, C.J., Faraone, S.V., et al. (2008). Motor coordination problems in children and adolescents with ADHD rated by parents and teachers: effects of age and gender. *Journal of Neural Transmission, 115,* 211–220.

Gadow, K.D. (1985). Prevalence and efficacy of stimulant drug use with mentally retarded children and youth. *Psychopharmacology Bulletin, 21,* 291–303.

Handen, B.L., Johnson, C.R., & Lubetsky, M. (2000). Efficacy of methylphenidate among children with autism and symptoms of attention-deficit hyperactivity disorder. *Journal of Autism and Developmental Disorders, 30,* 245–255.

Hoza, B., Pelham, W.E., Dobbs, J., Owens, J.S., & Pillow, D.R. (2002). Do boys with attention-deficit/hyperactivity disorder have positive illusory self-concepts? *Journal of Abnormal Psychology, 111,* 268–278.

Jahromi, L.B., Kasari, C.L., McCracken, J.T., Lee, L.S., Aman, M.G., McDougle, C.J., et al. (2009). Positive effects of methylphenidate on social communication and self-regulation in children with pervasive developmental disorders and hyperactivity. *Journal of Autism and Developmental Disorders, 39,* 395–404.

Lahey, B.B., Applegate, B., Barkley, R.A., Garfinkel, B., McBurnett, K., Kerdyk, L., et al. (1994). *DSM-IV* field trials for oppositional defiant disorder and conduct disorder in children and adolescents. *American Journal of Psychiatry, 151,* 1163–1171.

March, J.S., Swanson, J.M., Arnold, L.E., Hoza, B., Conners, C.K., Hinshaw, S.P., et al. (2000). Anxiety as a predictor and outcome variable in the Multimodal Treatment Study of Children with ADHD (MTA). *Journal of Abnormal Child Psychology, 28*(6), 527–541.

Mitsis, E.M., McKay, K.E., Schulz, K.P., Newcorn, J.H., & Halperin, J.M. (2000). Parent–teacher concordance for *DSM-IV* attention-deficit/hyperactivity disorder in a clinic-referred sample. *Child and Adolescent Psychiatry, 39,* 308–313.

Murray, D.W., Bussing, R., Fernandez, M., Wei, H., Garvan, C.W., Swanson, J.M., et al. (2009). Psychometric properties of teacher SKAMP ratings from a community sample. *Assessment, 16,* 193–208.

Reynolds, C.R., & Kamphouse, R.W. (1992). *BASC: Behavior Assessment System for Children manual.* Circle Pines, MN: American Guidance Service.

Sleator, E.K., Neumann, A., & Sprague, R.L. (1974). Hyperactive children: A continuous long-term placebo-controlled follow-up. *JAMA: The Journal of the American Medical Association, 229,* 316–317.

Shepperd, S., Doll, H., Gowers, S., James, A., Fazel, M., Fitzpatrick, R., et al. (2009). *Alternatives to inpatient mental health care for children and young people.* (Cochrane Database of Systematic Reviews No. CD006410)

Smith, B.H., Pelham, W.E., Jr., Gnagy, E., Molina, B., & Evans, S. (2000). The reliability, validity, and unique contributions of self-report by adolescents receiving treatment for attention-deficit/hyperactivity disorder. *Journal of Consulting and Clinical Psychology, 68,* 489–499.

Smucker, M.R., Craighead, W.E., Craighead, L.W., & Green, B.J. (1986). Normative and reliability data for the Children's Depression Inventory. *Journal of Abnormal Child Psychology, 14,* 25–39.

Swanson, J.M., Nolan, W., & Pelham, W.E. (1981). *The SNAP Rating Scale for the diagnosis of the attention deficit disorder.* (ERIC Document Reproduction Service No. ED217047)

Swedo, S.E., Henrietta, L.I.., Garvey, M., Mittleman, B., Allen, A.J., Perlmutter, S., et al. (1998). Pediatric autoimmune neuropsychiatric disorders associated with streptococcal infections: Clinical description of the first 50 cases. *American Journal of Psychiatry, 155,* 264–271.

van Gastel, W., & Ferdinand, R.F. (2008). Screening capacity of the Multidimensional Anxiety Scale for Children (MASC) for *DSM-IV* anxiety disorders. *Depression and Anxiety, 25,* 1046–1052.

Wechsler, D. (2003). *WISC–IV Technical and Interpretive Manual.* San Antonio, TX: Psychological Corporation.

Weyandt, L.L., Iwaszuk, W., Fulton, K., Ollerton, M., Beatty, N., Fouts, H., et al. (2003) The internal restlessness scale: Performance of college students with and without ADHD. *Journal of Learning Disabilities, 36*(4), 382–389.

Wolraich, M.L., Felice, M.E., &Drotar, D.D. (1996). *The classification of child and adolescent mental conditions in primary care: Diagnostic and Statistical Manual for Primary Care (DSM-PC) Child and Adolescent Version.* Elk Grove, IL, American Academy of Pediatrics.

Wolraich, M.L., Feurer, I.D., Hannah, J.N., Baumgartel, A., & Pinnock, T.Y. (1998). Obtaining systematic teacher reports of disruptive behavior disorders utilizing *DSM-IV. Journal of Abnormal Child Psychology, 26,* 141–152.

Woodcock, R., McGrew, K.S., & Mather, N. (2000). *Woodcock-Johnson III Tests of Achievement.* Itasca, IL: Riverside Publishing.

CHAPTER 5

Functional Impairments

Children and adolescents with attention-deficit/hyperactivity disorder (ADHD) typically experience significant impairment in one or more areas of functioning, including academic performance/achievement and social relationships with peers or adult authority figures. The fact that ADHD symptoms are associated with functional impairment is not surprising given that the *Diagnostic and Statistical Manual of Mental Disorders, Fourth Edition, Text Revision* (*DSM-IV-TR*; American Psychiatric Association [APA], 2000) criteria for this disorder require symptom-associated impairment in academic, social, or occupational functioning to make the diagnosis. Consideration of functional impairment is critically important because problems with academic and social functioning, rather than ADHD symptoms, often are the primary reason for referral in clinical and school settings. Furthermore, successful treatments are those strategies that lead not only to symptom reduction but also enhance academic and social outcomes.

The purpose of this chapter is to describe possible areas of impairment associated with ADHD, including academic skills and performance as well as relationships with peers and adult authority figures. Implications of functional impairment for assessment and intervention also are addressed.

Impairment in
Academic Skills and Performance

Children with ADHD typically exhibit a variety of difficulties that may compromise academic functioning. First, children with this disorder are frequently inattentive and exhibit significantly higher rates of off-task behavior relative to their classmates without ADHD (e.g., Abikoff et al., 2002; Vile Junod, DuPaul, Jitendra, Volpe, & Cleary, 2006). Rates of on-task behavior are particularly low when passive classroom activities (e.g., listening to teacher instruction, reading silently) are required (Vile Junod et al., 2006). In addition, the hyperactive/impulsive behaviors that may comprise ADHD (e.g., talking without permission, leaving the assigned area, bothering other students, interrupting teacher instruction) often lead to disruptive behaviors in the classroom and other school environments. Furthermore, 45%–84% of children with ADHD can be diagnosed with oppositional defiant disorder (ODD), wherein students may frequently disobey teacher commands and overtly defy school rules (Barkley, 2006). The combination of ADHD and disruptive behavior can interfere with learning for students with ADHD and their classmates.

Academic underachievement can be caused by deficits in academic skills, academic performance, or both. An academic skill deficit represents a lack of ability to learn a specific subject matter (e.g., reading), at least as the material is typically taught in a general education classroom. The more common term for an academic skill deficit is *learning disability*. Alternatively, an academic performance deficit is defined as a situation in which a student possesses the necessary ability but does not demonstrate this knowledge on a consistent basis under typical classroom conditions (e.g., by producing accurate independent seatwork). Although only about 30% of students with ADHD have academic skill deficits or learning disabilities (for review, see DuPaul & Stoner, 2003), most students with this disorder exhibit academic performance deficits related to underachievement.

ADHD symptoms appear to contribute to academic performance deficits in at least three ways (DuPaul & Stoner, 2003). First, inattention and behavior control difficulties can compromise a student's availability for learning (e.g., missing teacher instruction due to inattention) and thus lead to academic underachievement (Silver, 1990). Second, a lack of attention to academic materials may lead to poor performance on written assignments, even though children may possess the necessary skills to complete the assignment accurately. Finally, academic performance may be deleteriously affected by impulsive behavior as well as inefficient and inconsistent problem-solving strategies (Douglas, 1980).

The academic achievement difficulties of children and adolescents with ADHD have been demonstrated in several ways. On average, students with ADHD score between 10 to 30 points lower than classmates without ADHD on norm-referenced, standardized achievement tests (e.g., Barkley, DuPaul, & McMurray, 1990; Brock & Knapp, 1996; Fischer, Barkley, Fletcher, & Smallish, 1990). In fact, a recent meta-analysis indicated a moderate to large effect size difference in achievement scores for children with ADHD relative to typically developing peers (Frazier, Youngstrom, Glutting, & Watkins, 2007). Approximately 20%–30% of students with ADHD also have a specific learning disability in reading, math, or writing (DuPaul & Stoner, 2003; Semrud-Clikeman et al., 1992). ADHD symptoms (i.e., inattention, impulsivity, hyperactivity) have been found to be significant predictors of concurrent and future academic difficulties (e.g., performance on achievement tests, report card grades, teacher ratings of educational functioning). The relationship between ADHD symptoms and achievement outcomes is evident for both referred (DuPaul et al., 2004) and nonreferred (Fergusson & Horwood, 1995) samples. As a result, students with ADHD are at higher risk for grade retention, placement in special education classrooms, and dropping out from high school (e.g., Fischer et al., 1990). Fewer students with ADHD go on to postsecondary education relative to similarly achieving classmates without ADHD (Mannuzza, Gittelman-Klein, Bessler, Malloy, & LaPadula, 1993). Thus, poor educational functioning throughout the school years is a frequent outcome for students with ADHD.

A dual pathway model to explain the relationship between ADHD symptoms and academic achievement difficulties has been examined in several studies (e.g., Fergusson & Horwood, 1995; Rapport, Scanlan, & Denny, 1999). For example, Rapport and colleagues proposed both cognitive and behavioral mediators of the effects of ADHD on achievement. The cognitive pathway is hypothesized to mediate the impact of ADHD on achievement through vigilance and memory deficits, while the behavioral pathway mediates the impact of ADHD on achievement via disruptive classroom behavior. Two other studies have extended this model by examining variables that may account for the connection between ADHD and achievement problems in mathematics and reading (DuPaul et al., 2004; Volpe et al., 2006). The results of these investigations indicated that important classroom behaviors (e.g., motivation, study skills, academic engagement) acted as mediators of the effects of ADHD and prior achievement on current achievement. Thus, the relationship between ADHD symptoms and achievement is complex, implying that practitioners and researchers should not expect that one specific intervention focusing on a single target will be sufficient in ameliorating academic difficulties.

A study examining the effects of academic interventions on achievement of elementary school students further illustrates the pervasiveness and magnitude of academic impairments experienced by individuals with ADHD (for details, see DuPaul et al., 2006; Jitendra et al., 2007). Participants in this study included 87 children who met *DSM-IV-TR* criteria for ADHD and 37 typically developing classmates who did not exhibit academic or behavioral difficulties. All children were between the ages of 7 and 10 years old and were placed in first-through fourth-grade general education classrooms. Prior to intervention, several measures were used to document the degree to which students with ADHD experienced classroom and academic difficulties.

All participants were observed for 20 minutes each in their reading and math classes to assess the frequency of on- and off-task behavior. The Behavioral Observation of Students in Schools (BOSS; Shapiro, 2003) coding system was used. The BOSS focuses on five behaviors including active on-task (e.g., reading aloud, answering teacher questions), passive on-task (e.g., listening to teacher instructions, reading silently), off-task motor (e.g., fidgeting, leaving seat without permission), off-task verbal (e.g., talking without permission, making noises), and off-task passive (e.g., not looking at the teacher during instruction). Children with ADHD exhibited significantly higher rates of all three off-task behaviors as well as significantly lower rates of passive on-task behavior relative to classmates without ADHD in both math and reading (see Figures 5.1 and 5.2). Between-group differences were

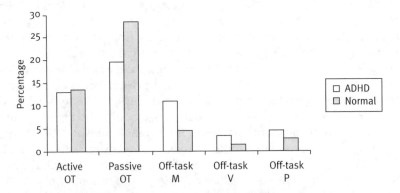

Figure 5.1.   Percentage of observation intervals on the Behavioral Observation of Students in Schools (BOSS; Shapiro, 2003) coding system for children with and without attention-deficit/hyperactivity disorder (ADHD) during math class. Behaviors included active on-task (active OT), passive on-task (passive OT), off-task motor (off-task M), off-task verbal (off-task V), and off-task passive (off-task P).

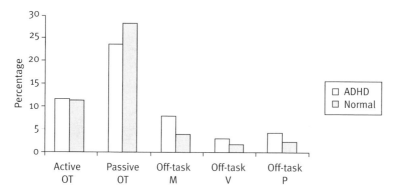

Figure 5.2. Percentage of observation intervals on the Behavioral Observation of Students in Schools (BOSS; Shapiro, 2003) coding system for children with and without attention-deficit/hyperactivity disorder (ADHD) during reading class. Behaviors included active on-task (active OT), passive on-task (passive OT), off-task motor (off-task M), off-task verbal (off-task V), and off-task passive (off-task P).

relatively large (i.e., more than 0.5 standard deviation units). Interestingly, groups did not differ in frequency of active on-task behavior suggesting that children with ADHD can be as engaged as their classmates provided that active responding is required.

The reading and math achievement of this sample was evaluated using the Woodcock-Johnson III Tests of Achievement (Woodcock, McGrew, & Mather, 2000). Children with ADHD received standard scores in broad reading and broad math that were significantly lower than scores obtained by their peers without ADHD (see Figure 5.3). In fact, these groups differed by at least one standard

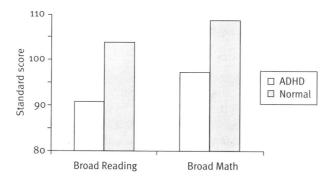

Figure 5.3. Broad Reading and Broad Math standard scores on the Woodcock-Johnson III Tests of Achievement (Woodcock, McGrew, & Mather, 2000) for students with and without attention-deficit/hyperactivity disorder (ADHD).

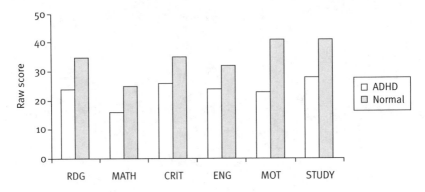

Figure 5.4. Raw scores on the Academic Competency Evaluation Scale (ACES; DiPerna &
Elliott, 2000) for students with and without attention-deficit/hyperactivity disorder
(ADHD). Subscales include Reading (RDG), Math, Critical Thinking (CRIT), Engagement
(ENG), Motivation (MOT), and Study Skills (STUDY).

deviation, indicating clinically significant impairment in academic
achievement for the ADHD group.

Teachers were asked to provide ratings of students' academic
skills and academic enabling behaviors (e.g., study skills and motivation) using the Academic Competence Evaluation Scale (ACES;
DiPerna & Elliott, 2000). The ACES includes six subscales: Reading,
Math, Critical Thinking, Engagement, Motivation, and Study Skills.
Students with ADHD were rated significantly lower than classmates
on all six dimensions (see Figure 5.4). These differences were quite
large, ranging from 2 to 3 standard deviations. Clearly, teachers viewed
students with ADHD as having multiple academic and behavioral
impairments relative to typically developing classmates.

Association Between
ADHD and Learning Disabilities

Children with ADHD not only experience academic performance
deficits, but a significant percentage of individuals with this disorder
have demonstrable skill deficits in one or more academic subject areas
(e.g., reading, math). In fact, approximately 30% of students with
ADHD also have a learning disability (DuPaul & Stoner, 2003; Semrud-
Clikeman et al., 1992). Furthermore, students with ADHD make up a
significant percentage of children identified for special education services because of a learning disability, ranging from 20.2% (Schnoes,
Reid, Wagner, & Marder, 2006) to 25% (Forness & Kavale, 2001). It is
unclear whether ADHD symptoms "cause" skill deficits or vice versa,

particularly because no study has adequately investigated this issue. Studies that have employed structural equation modeling have demonstrated that ADHD-related behaviors (primarily inattention) have a strong, negative impact on later academic achievement (e.g., Rowe & Rowe, 1992). Although the converse (i.e., reading difficulties may lead to inattention) may also be true, this directional relationship typically is weaker than the negative impact of ADHD symptoms on achievement. Regardless of the putative causal direction of this relationship, it is clear that children with ADHD are at higher than average risk for learning disabilities. This possibility must be taken into account when assessing and treating individuals with ADHD.

Impairment in Relationships with Peers and Authority Figures

Children and adolescents with ADHD often have significant difficulty developing and maintaining positive relationships with peers, parents, and teachers (Barkley, 2006; DuPaul & Stoner, 2003). As was the case for academic achievement problems, social relationship difficulties may be due to social skills deficits (i.e., individuals lack age-appropriate behaviors in their repertoire) and/or social performance deficits (i.e., individuals possess the requisite social skills but do not perform them at appropriate or required times). Although children with ADHD may lack specific social skills, it seems that most of their social relationship difficulties are due to performance deficits (Barkley, 2006). It should be noted that social performance deficits associated with ADHD are exacerbated by the presence of a comorbid externalizing disorder (i.e., ODD or conduct disorder) presumably due to the aggression and noncompliance associated with the latter conditions (Booster, DuPaul, Eiraldi, & Power, 2009).

The symptomatic behaviors of ADHD appear to lead to social performance deficits in several ways. First, children with ADHD may not consistently follow the implicit rules of reciprocal conversation (Stroes, Alberts, & van der Meere, 2003). A child with ADHD is likely to interrupt during conversation, not listen closely to what others are saying, and respond in an irrelevant fashion (i.e., talk about something that is not germane to the conversation topic). Second, students with ADHD may enter ongoing peer activities (e.g., games, conversations) in an abrupt, impulsive manner, thereby disrupting the activity to a significant degree (DuPaul & Stoner, 2003). Peers may choose to exclude the child with ADHD from activities as a result. Third, children with this disorder are more likely than their classmates without ADHD to behave in a verbally or physically aggressive manner, presumably due to their problems with impulse control (Barkley, 2006). Finally, given this combination of social relationship difficulties, several studies have indicated that children with ADHD are less well liked, more often rejected, and have fewer friends than their peers without ADHD (e.g., Hoza et al., 2005). Furthermore, as they grow older, children with ADHD and related behavior disorders may befriend each other and form deviant peer groups that could lead to an escalation of delinquent and conduct disordered behavior (Patterson, Reid, & Dishion, 1992).

ADHD symptoms not only disrupt the development of appropriate peer relationships but also deleteriously affect children's interactions with family members and adult authority figures (e.g., teachers). A child's inattention problems and noncompliance often are associated with significantly higher levels of parental stress, particularly among mothers (Johnston & Mash, 2001). In addition, parents of children with ADHD are more likely to use higher-order controls (e.g., punishment) to control behavior. This may lead to more frequent negative—even aggressive—interactions in these families than in families of typically developing children (Barkley, 2006). Frequently, noncompliant and negative interactions extend to teacher–child relationships as well (DuPaul & Stoner, 2003).

Implications of Impairment for Assessment

There are at least two compelling reasons why assessment of functional impairment must be included in the comprehensive evaluation of children and adolescents suspected of having ADHD. First, as articulated earlier in this chapter, symptoms of this disorder are frequently associated with clinically significant difficulties in academic and/or social functioning. Second, the percentage of children meeting criteria for ADHD varies significantly when impairment is or is not considered as part of the diagnosis (Gathje, Lewandowski, & Gordon, 2008). In fact, Gathje and colleagues found that symptoms and impairment are only moderately correlated and thus represent distinct constructs that must be measured independently. As a result, the diagnostic evaluation of ADHD should include reliable and valid measures of academic and social functioning (DuPaul & Stoner, 2003; Pelham, Fabiano, & Massetti, 2005).

Measures are available to evaluate impairment at both global and specific levels. These indices can be used to establish whether clinically significant levels of impairment are associated with ADHD symptoms. Furthermore, areas of impairment should be assessed in a continuous fashion, particularly when interventions are first implemented (i.e., to evaluate treatment effects on academic and social functioning).

Several measures of general impairment are available. These include the Columbia Impairment Rating Scale (Bird et al., 1993), Children's Global Assessment of Functioning (Bird, Canino, Rubio-Stipec, & Ribera, 1987), Clinical Global Impression–Severity (Guy, 2000), Impairment Rating Scale (Fabiano et al., 2006), and Child and Adolescent Functional Assessment Scale (Hodges, Doucette-Gates, & Liao, 1999). In the case of the Clinical Global Impression–Severity, clinicians document children's overall level of functioning based on information received from parents and/or teachers as well as review of archival material (e.g., school records). Typically, an overall score is awarded to place children's functioning at one point in a continuum ranging from low to superior functioning. The Impairment Rating Scale can also be completed by a clinician but is constructed for parent and/or teacher respondents. Rather than one overall impairment rating, the Impairment Rating Scale asks respondents to indicate the degree to which ADHD symptoms are associated with impairment in several areas including academic/school performance and interactions with others.

Although these general measures of impairment/functioning have adequate reliability and validity, they have several limitations. First, global indices typically rely on a clinician to make a summary judgment based on information gleaned from one or more primary sources (e.g., parent, teacher, archival information). As such, considerable subjectivity may be involved in the scoring process. Second, a global rating of impairment may obscure important differences in functioning levels across areas of impairment. For example, some children with ADHD may present with social relationship difficulties but not academic underachievement (or vice versa). Thus, a single score cannot represent potential differences in functioning across areas. Third, a similar limitation is that because general impairment indices are global, direct measurement of specific subareas within each area of functioning is not possible. Stated differently, a global impairment score does not indicate what specific social and/or academic difficulties children are experiencing. For example, some children with ADHD may have difficulty interacting with peers in unstructured settings (e.g., playground) and may manifest this difficulty by behaving aggressively. Other children may also have difficulties interacting with peers but exhibit this in structured settings (e.g., classroom), particularly with respect to cooperating with group rules. Thus, a comprehensive assessment approach should include specific measures of academic and social functioning.

Assessment of Academic Skills and Performance

Academic skills and performance can be assessed using direct measures, indirect measures, or their combination. Direct measurement of academic skills involves administering a test to children to evaluate their level of skill in reading, math, or other academic subject areas. Traditionally, norm-referenced achievement tests such as the Woodcock-Johnson III or the Wechsler Individual Achievement Test (Wechsler, 1992) have been used for this purpose. These norm-referenced tests have well-established psychometric properties and provide standard scores that indicate student performance relative to a norm group (typically based on grade or age). Furthermore, tests such as the Woodcock-Johnson III and Wechsler Individual Achievement Test include specific subscales related to skill areas within math, reading, or other academic subjects. Thus, test scores can be used to 1) determine whether individual children are functioning at expected levels (or below or above expected levels) and 2) delineate specific areas of academic strength and weakness. Unfortunately, norm-referenced achievement tests are rather limited for making instructional or intervention decisions because they include only a few items per grade level, are not tied directly to the curriculum being taught, and may suffer from practice effects if used on a periodic basis to assess change over time (e.g., to assess treatment effects).

Another way to directly assess academic skills is to use curriculum-based measurement (CBM; Shinn, 1998). CBM involves constructing brief 1- to 5-minute probes of reading or math skills using items directly taken from a student's instructional curriculum. Generic math and reading probes are also available (http://www.aimsweb.com). Thus, CBM data can quickly and efficiently provide information relevant to student placement in curriculum materials (i.e., help teachers match instructional materials to student skill level), areas of relative strength and weakness, and progress over time as a function of instructional intervention. Given the myriad of potential uses and relative cost and time efficiency, CBM is preferred over norm-referenced achievement testing in most cases.

Permanent products can also be used to directly assess academic performance. For example, in-class written assignments can be examined to determine the degree to which students have completed the assignment as well as the accuracy of responses. Percentages of completion and accuracy on assignments can be compared to classmates without ADHD or to a class average to determine the degree to which a specific student may be underperforming or overperforming. Clinicians can also examine products over time to gauge the degree to which students are inconsistent or variable in their work productivity and accuracy. Frequently, children with ADHD exhibit variable performance over time with respect to schoolwork. Percentages of completion and accuracy can also be used to evaluate the effects of treatment, including medication (e.g., Rapport & Denney, 2000).

Academic skills and performance can also be assessed using indirect measures, primarily teacher ratings. The Academic Performance Rating Scale (DuPaul, Rapport, & Perriello, 1991) is a brief measure that teachers can complete to indicate student performance in reading, math, writing, and other academic skills and behaviors (e.g., organizational skills). The Academic Performance Rating Scale can be used as either an initial index of impairment during the diagnostic evaluation or serve as a brief measure to monitor progress as a function of treatment. A more comprehensive teacher rating of academic performance is the ACES, which includes subscales related to academic skills in math, reading, and critical thinking as well as subscales tapping "academic enablers" including study skills, motivation, and engagement (see Figure 5.4). It is a norm-referenced instrument that indicates teacher perception of student status in each key area relative to classmates. Because of the length of this measure, it may be less efficient than the briefer Academic Performance Rating Scale as a progress monitoring measure.

Assessment of Social Behavior and Peer Relationships

The social behavior and peer relationships of children and adolescents with ADHD can be assessed with both direct and indirect methods. Direct measurement of social behavior typically involves observation of peer interactions in classroom or playground settings. Several observation codes have been developed for this purpose, including the ADHD Social Observation Code (Gadow, Sprafkin, & Nolan, 1996) and the Early Screening Project coding system (Walker, Severson, & Feil, 1995). Typically, brief (15–20 minutes) observations of child interactions with peers are conducted to determine the percentage of observation intervals when prosocial vs. antisocial (e.g., aggressive) behavior occurs. In addition to being a direct measure of social behavior, two additional advantages of observations are the assessment of peer interactions in context (i.e., in response to events in the social environment) and the opportunity to compare a target child's behavior to peers without ADHD who are interacting in the same social environment. The primary disadvantage of conducting observations is the time involved in collecting these data.

Indirect methods for assessing social behavior include social skills rating scales completed by parents, teachers, and target students, as well as sociometric indices or peer ratings. Several social behavior rating scales are commercially available, including the Social Skills Improvement System (SSIS; Elliott & Gresham, 2008) and the Walker-McConnell Social Behavior Scale (Walker & McConnell, 1988). As is the case for norm-referenced achievement measures, the chief advantage of these rating scales is that they provide scores that indicate a target student's status relative to others of the same age and gender. Furthermore, rating scales provide clinicians with parent, teacher, and student perspectives about social behavior in both home and school settings. An additional advantage of the SSIS is the inclusion of rating scale measures that tie directly to a broader intervention system, including both schoolwide and classroom-based interventions. Sociometric measures and peer ratings involve children either nominating peers as preferred or nonpreferred playmates or rating the social behavior of their classmates (e.g., Asher & Dodge, 1986). Concerns about protecting confidentiality and obtaining parent permission typically relegate sociometric and peer ratings to research contexts.

Implications of Impairment for Treatment

As discussed in this chapter, children and adolescents with ADHD may experience functional impairments in several key areas, chiefly with respect to academic achievement and peer relationships. It is particularly important to consider functional impairment in treatment planning because the type and level of impairment independently predicts service use by families of children with ADHD above and beyond the severity of symptomatic behaviors (Sawyer et al., 2004). Unfortunately, although psychotropic medications (chiefly the stimulants) are frequently effective in reducing the core symptoms of this disorder, this treatment typically has minimal impact on associated impairments, particularly over the long term (e.g., Jensen et al., 2007). The other primary treatment for ADHD—behavior modification—can more directly address functional impairments, especially those in the social domain. Nevertheless, a comprehensive treatment approach (as described more fully in Chapters 6 and 8) will include interventions that directly target areas of impairment (i.e., go beyond symptom reduction). Specific strategies can be used to enhance academic skills/performance, improve social behavior and peer relationships, and facilitate better interactions with authority figures.

Strategies to Enhance Academic Skills/Performance

Students with ADHD often experience difficulties with academic achievement and development of core reading and math skills (DuPaul & Stoner, 2003; Hinshaw, 1992). Thus, interventions directly addressing academic deficits are necessary. Although academic interventions for students with ADHD have not been as widely studied as behavioral treatments for this population, recent studies have provided initial support for academic remediation strategies. The results of single-subject research design studies support the efficacy of computer-assisted instruction (Clarfield & Stoner, 2005; Mautone, DuPaul, & Jitendra, 2005; Ota & DuPaul, 2002), classwide peer tutoring (DuPaul, Ervin, Hook, & McGoey, 1998), home-based parent tutoring (Hook & DuPaul, 1999) or homework support (Power, Karustis, & Habboushe, 2001), self-regulated strategy for written expression (Reid & Lienemann, 2006), and directed notetaking (Evans, Pelham, & Grudberg, 1995) in enhancing specific areas of academic performance. These strategies are discussed in greater detail in Chapter 8.

Beyond their positive impact on achievement, academic interventions also have several advantages as a treatment for students with ADHD. First, most academic strategies emphasize the modification of antecedent events (e.g., instruction and/or task presentation) that may precede problematic inattentive or impulsive behavior. Thus, in terms of behavior management, academic interventions may be considered proactive or preventive. As a result, a second advantage of academic remediation strategies is that they may lead to changes in problematic behavior. Stated differently, improvements in academic performance may lead to or be associated with enhancement of behavior control. In fact, effect sizes for behavior change associated with academic interventions are very similar to effect sizes obtained for behavior modification strategies like contingency management (DuPaul & Eckert, 1997).

Thus, in some cases, academic interventions may serve the dual purpose of improving academic skills and reducing inattentive behaviors. Finally, many of the academic strategies studied thus far involve the use of mediators (e.g., peers, parents, computers) beyond an exclusive reliance on classroom teachers. The use of multiple mediators may enhance the acceptability and feasibility of classroom-based treatment by reducing the burden on teachers.

Strategies to Enhance Social Behavior and Peer Relationships

Children and adolescents with ADHD often experience difficulties with peer relationships, including making and keeping friends (Barkley, 2006; Weyandt, 2007). As discussed previously, it appears that peer relationship difficulties are secondary to performance rather than skill deficits (Barkley, 2006). Unfortunately, social performance deficits are more difficult to ameliorate than skills problems for two reasons. First, most currently available social relationship interventions target deficits in skills rather than performance. Furthermore, because social performance problems occur across settings (e.g., classroom, playground, neighborhood), interventions addressing these difficulties must be implemented by a variety of individuals in a cross-situational fashion.

Not surprisingly, interventions that target social knowledge and the acquisition of prosocial behaviors in group therapy formats (i.e., "traditional" social skills training) have not been found to lead to durable changes in interpersonal functioning in "real-world" environments. Although impressive gains in conversation skills, problem solving, and anger control have been obtained during training sessions themselves, rarely do these improvements continue once the child leaves the therapy room (DuPaul & Eckert, 1994; Gresham, 2002).

The lack of maintenance and generalization of traditional social skills training has led to proposals for a more comprehensive approach to social relationship intervention for children with disruptive behavior disorders (for a review of social skills strategies, see Gresham, 2002). For example, Sheridan (1995) developed the Tough Kids Social Skills program for use in school settings, and Sheridan and colleagues (1996) have established preliminary empirical support for using the program with students with ADHD. This program includes three possible levels of social skills training including small group, classwide, and schoolwide. Although all three training levels may be helpful for students with ADHD, it is likely that children with this disorder will require small group training given their protracted relationship difficulties.

Relatively few studies of social relationship interventions for children with ADHD have been conducted, especially in school settings. Most prior investigations of social skills training have been conducted in outpatient clinic settings with minimal school outcome data beyond teacher ratings. Results of these clinic-based studies are equivocal with respect to efficacy (e.g., Antshel & Remer, 2003; Frankel, Myatt, & Cantwell, 1995; Pfiffner & McBurnett, 1997). Outcomes of these interventions are enhanced when specific strategies are included to program for maintenance and generalization of effects. For example, peers without ADHD could be involved in all phases of a social relationship intervention to encourage generality of outcomes. First, peers can participate in role-play activities and provide feedback to target students, in essence serving in a "co-therapist" role. Second, peers could serve as social skills "tutors" in the natural environment by prompting and reinforcing the enactment of social behaviors that have been targeted in the training sessions. Cunningham and Cunningham (2006) have developed a student-mediated conflict resolution program that involves peers acting as playground monitors. Cunningham and Cunningham found that peer-mediated conflict resolution led to schoolwide reductions in playground violence and negative interactions.

Strategies to Improve Interactions with Family Members and Authority Figures

Relationships between children with ADHD and their family members, particularly parents, can be affected by the symptomatic behaviors associated with this disorder. Specifically, family life with a child with ADHD is characterized by high levels of parental stress and frequent, negative, coercive interactions among family members (Johnston & Mash, 2001; Patterson et al., 1992). Furthermore, inattentive, impulsive, and/or noncompliant behavior in the classroom can strain relationships between teachers and their students with ADHD (DuPaul & Stoner, 2003). The primary intervention approach to addressing family difficulties has been the use of behavioral parent training in a strategic fashion to reduce child noncompliance and aggression (for more details, see Chapters 6 and 7). In similar fashion, classroom teachers can employ positive reinforcement, token economy, and related behavioral strategies to enhance student attention to academic demands and compliance with rules (for more details, see Chapter 8). As a function of enhanced child compliance and improved behavior, interactions between children with ADHD and authority figures are improved markedly. Furthermore, levels of parent and teacher stress are reduced (Barkley, 2006). For adolescents with ADHD, families can be taught to engage in problem-solving and communication training in order to improve the quality of interactions among family members (Robin & Foster, 1989). In fact, Barkley and colleagues (1992) found problem-solving and communication training to improve parent reports of teen home behavior, especially when combined with behavioral contracting procedures.

Conclusions

ADHD is frequently associated with clinically significant impairment in child and adolescent functioning, particularly in the areas of academic achievement and relationships with peers and authority figures. In fact, *DSM-IV-TR* criteria require symptoms to be associated with impairment in at least one setting. In the area of academic performance, individuals with this disorder typically obtain low average to below average achievement scores, are at higher than average risk for grade retention and/or receipt of special education services, and may be at significant risk for school dropout (Barkley, 2006). Furthermore, students with ADHD are less likely to obtain postsecondary education; of those who do attend college, there is a higher than average risk for noncompletion of degree (Barkley, Murphy, & Fischer, 2008). Functioning in the social domain is similarly affected, wherein children with ADHD have fewer friends and experience greater levels of peer rejection than their typically developing peers (McQuade & Hoza, 2008). High frequency and severity of verbal aggression, physical fighting, and/or noncompliance with adult rules and commands are associated with disrupted relationships with peers, siblings, parents, and teachers (Barkley, 2006).

Given the high risk for significant impairment, primary care physicians and educators should collaborate to implement assessment and treatment strategies that go beyond a focus on symptomatic behaviors and include attention to academic and social functioning. Thus, a comprehensive evaluation of ADHD should include both general and specific measures of impairment. In similar fashion, treatment programs should include strategies that directly address areas of impairment because functional impairments are not appreciably affected by psychotropic medication. Once an intervention plan is implemented, assessment data should be collected periodically to evaluate not only whether treatment has led to improvements in symptomatic behaviors, but also to gauge whether intervention provides concomitant enhancement of academic and social functioning.

References

Abikoff, H.B., Jensen, P.S., Arnold, L.L.E., Hoza, B., Hechtman, L., Pollack, S., et al. (2002). Observed classroom behavior of children with ADHD: Relationship to gender and comorbidity. *Journal of Abnormal Child Psychology, 20,* 349–359.

American Psychiatric Association. (2000). *Diagnostic and statistical manual of mental disorders* (4th ed., Text rev.). Washington, DC: Author.

Antshel, K.M., & Remer, R. (2003). Social skills training in children with attention deficit hyperactivity disorder: A randomized-controlled clinical trial. *Journal of Clinical Child and Adolescent Psychology, 32,* 153–165.

Asher, S.R., & Dodge, K.A. (1986). Identifying children who are rejected by their peers. *Developmental Psychology, 22,* 444–449.

Barkley, R.A. (Ed.). (2006). *Attention-deficit/hyperactivity disorder: A handbook for diagnosis and treatment* (3rd ed.). New York: Guilford Press.

Barkley, R.A., DuPaul, G.J., & McMurray, M.B. (1990). A comprehensive evaluation of attention deficit disorder with and without hyperactivity as defined by research criteria. *Journal of Consulting and Clinical Psychology, 58,* 775–789.

Barkley, R.A., Guevremont, D.C., Anastopoulos, A.D., & Fletcher, K.E. (1992). A comparison of three family therapy programs for treating family conflicts in adolescents with attention-deficit hyperactivity disorder. *Journal of Consulting and Clinical Psychology, 60,* 450–462.

Barkley, R.A., Murphy, K.R., & Fischer, M. (2008). *ADHD in adults: What the science says.* New York: Guilford Press.

Bird, H.R., Canino, G., Rubio-Stipec, M., & Ribera, J.C. (1987). Further measures of the psychometric properties of the Children's Global Assessment Scale. *Archives of General Psychiatry, 44,* 821–824.

Bird, H.R., Shaffer, D., Fisher, P., Gould, M.S., Staghezza, B., Chen, J.Y., et al. (1993). The Columbia Impairment Scale (CIS): Pilot findings on a measure of global impairment for children and adolescents. *International Journal of Methods in Psychiatric Research, 3,* 167–176.

Booster, G.D., DuPaul, G.J., Eiraldi, R., & Power, T.J. (2009). *Functional impairments in children with ADHD: Unique effects of comorbid status and ADHD subtype.* Manuscript submitted for publication.

Brock, S.W., & Knapp, P.K. (1996). Reading comprehension abilities of children with attention-deficit/hyperactivity disorder. *Journal of Attention Disorders, 1,* 173–186.

Clarfield, J., & Stoner, G. (2005). The effects of computerized reading instruction on the academic performance of students identified with ADHD. *School Psychology Review, 34,* 246–254.

Cunningham, C.E., & Cunningham, L.J. (2006). Student-mediated conflict resolution programs. In R.A. Barkley (Ed.), *Attention-deficit hyperactivity disorder: A handbook for diagnosis and treatment* (3rd ed., pp. 590–607). New York: Guilford Press.

DiPerna, J.C., & Elliott, S.N. (2000). *Academic Competence Evaluation Scales.* San Antonio, TX: The Psychological Corporation.

Douglas, V.I. (1980). Higher mental processes in hyperactive children: Implications for training. In R. Knights & D. Bakker (Eds.), *Treatment of hyperactive and learning disordered children* (pp. 65–92). Baltimore: University Park Press.

DuPaul, G.J., & Eckert, T.L. (1994). The effects of social skills curricula: Now you see them, now you don't. *School Psychology Quarterly, 9,* 113–132.

DuPaul, G.J., & Eckert, T.L. (1997). School-based interventions for children with attention-deficit/hyperactivity disorder: A meta-analysis. *School Psychology Review, 26,* 5–27.

DuPaul, G.J., Ervin, R.A., Hook, C.L., & McGoey, K.E. (1998). Peer tutoring for children with attention deficit hyperactivity disorder: Effects on classroom behavior and academic performance. *Journal of Applied Behavior Analysis, 31,* 579–592.

DuPaul, G.J., Jitendra, A.K., Volpe, R.J., Tresco, K.E., Lutz, J.G., Vile Junod, R.E., et al. (2006). Consultation-based academic interventions for children with ADHD: Effects on reading and mathematics achievement. *Journal of Abnormal Child Psychology, 34,* 633–646.

DuPaul, G.J., Rapport, M.D., & Perriello, L.M. (1991). Teacher ratings of academic skills: The development of the Academic Performance Rating Scale. *School Psychology Review, 20,* 284–300.

DuPaul, G.J., & Stoner, G. (2003). *ADHD in the schools: Assessment and intervention strategies* (2nd ed.). New York: Guilford Press.

DuPaul, G.J., Volpe, R.J., Jitendra, A.K., Lutz, J.G., Lorah, K.S., & Gruber, R. (2004). Elementary school students with AD/HD: Predictors of academic achievement. *Journal of School Psychology, 42,* 285–301.

Elliott, S.N., & Gresham, F.M. (2008). *SSIS (Social Skills Improvement System) Rating Scales.* San Antonio, TX: Pearson.

Evans, S.W., Pelham, W., & Grudberg, M.V. (1995). The efficacy of notetaking to improve behavior and comprehension of adolescents with attention deficit hyperactivity disorder. *Exceptionality, 5,* 1–17.

Fabiano, G.A., Pelham, W.E., Jr., Waschbusch, D.A., Gnagy, E.M., Lahey, B.B., Chronis, A.M., et al. (2006). A practical measure of impairment: Psychometric properties of the Impairment Rating Scale in samples of children with attention deficit hyperactivity disorder and two school-based samples. *Journal of Clinical Child and Adolescent Psychology, 35,* 369–385.

Fergusson, D.M., & Horwood, L.J. (1995). Early disruptive behavior, IQ, and later school achievement and delinquent behavior. *Journal of Abnormal Child Psychology, 23,* 183–199.

Fischer, M., Barkley, R.A., Fletcher, K., & Smallish, L. (1990). The adolescent outcome of hyperactive children diagnosed by research criteria: II. Academic, attentional, and neuropsychological status. *Journal of Consulting and Clinical Psychology, 58,* 580–588.

Forness, S.R., & Kavale, K.A. (2001). ADHD and a return to the medical model of special education. *Education and Treatment of Children, 24,* 224–247.

Frankel, F., Myatt, R., & Cantwell, D.P. (1995). Training outpatient boys to conform with the social ecology of popular peers: Effects on parent and teacher ratings. *Journal of Clinical Child Psychology, 24,* 300–310.

Frazier, T.W., Youngstrom, E.A., Glutting, J.J., & Watkins, M.W. (2007). ADHD and achievement: Meta-analysis of the child, adolescent, and adult literatures and concomitant study with college students. *Journal of Learning Disabilities, 40,* 49–65.

Gadow, K.D., Sprafkin, J., & Nolan, E.E. (1996). *ADHD School Observation Code.* Stony Brook, NY: Checkmate Plus.

Gathje, R.A., Lewandowski, L.J., & Gordon, M. (2008). The role of impairment in the diagnosis of ADHD. *Journal of Attention Disorders, 11,* 529–537.

Gresham, F.M. (2002). Teaching social skills to high-risk children and youth: Preventive and remedial strategies. In M.R. Shinn, H.M. Walker, & G. Stoner (Eds.), *Interventions for academic and behavior problems II: Preventive and remedial approaches* (2nd ed., pp. 403–432). Washington, DC: National Association of School Psychologists.

Guy, W. (2000). Clinical Global Impression (CGI) scale. In A.J. Rush, M.B. First, & D. Blacker (Eds.), *Handbook of psychiatric measures*. Washington, DC: American Psychiatric Publishing.

Hinshaw, S.P. (1992). Academic underachievement, attention deficits, and aggression: Comorbidity and implications for intervention. *Journal of Consulting and Clinical Psychology, 60*, 893–903.

Hodges, K., Doucette-Gates, A., & Liao, Q. (1999). The relationship between the Child and Adolescent Functional Assessment Scale (CAFAS) and indicators of functioning. *Journal of Child and Family Studies, 8*, 109–122.

Hook, C.L., & DuPaul, G.J. (1999). Parent tutoring for students with attention deficit hyperactivity disorder: Effects on reading at home and school. *School Psychology Review, 28*, 60–75.

Hoza, B., Gerdes, A.C., Mrug, S., Hinshaw, S.P., Bukowski, W.M., Gold, J.A., et al. (2005). Peer-assessed outcomes in the Multimodal Treatment Study of Children with Attention Deficit Hyperactivity Disorder. *Journal of Clinical Child and Adolescent Psychology, 34*, 74–86.

Jensen, P.S., Arnold, E., Swanson, J.M., Vitiello, B., Abikoff, H.B., Greenhill, L.L., et al. (2007). 3-year follow-up of the NIMH MTA study. *Journal of the American Academy of Child and Adolescent Psychiatry, 46*, 989–1002.

Jitendra, A.K., DuPaul, G.J., Volpe, R.J., Tresco, K.E., Vile Junod, R.E., Lutz, J.G., et al. (2007). Consultation-based academic intervention for children with attention deficit hyperactivity disorder: School functioning outcomes. *School Psychology Review, 36*, 217–236.

Johnston, C., & Mash, E.J. (2001). Families of children with attention-deficit/hyperactivity disorder: Review and recommendations for future research. *Clinical Child and Family Psychology Review, 4*, 183–207.

Mannuzza, S., Gittelman-Klein, R., Bessler, A., Malloy, P., & LaPadula, M. (1993). Adult outcome of hyperactive boys: Educational achievement, occupational rank, and psychiatric status. *Archives of General Psychiatry, 50*, 565–576.

Mautone, J.A., DuPaul, G.J., & Jitendra, A.K. (2005). The effects of computer-assisted instruction on the mathematics performance and classroom behavior of children with attention-deficit/hyperactivity disorder. *Journal of Attention Disorders, 8*, 301–312.

McQuade, J.D., & Hoza, B. (2008). Peer problems in attention deficit hyperactivity disorder: Current status and future directions. *Developmental Disabilities Research Reviews, 14*, 320–324.

Ota, K.R., & DuPaul, G.J. (2002). Task engagement and mathematics performance in children with attention deficit hyperactivity disorder: Effects of supplemental computer instruction. *School Psychology Quarterly, 17*, 242–257.

Patterson, G.R., Reid, J.B., & Dishion, T.J. (1992). *Antisocial boys*. Eugene, OR: Castalia.

Pelham, W.E., Jr., Fabiano, G.A., & Massetti, G.M. (2005). Evidence-based assessment of attention deficit hyperactivity disorders in children and adolescents. *Journal of Clinical Child and Adolescent Psychology, 34*, 449–476.

Pfiffner, L.J., & McBurnett, K. (1997). Social skills training with parent generalization: Treatment effects for children with attention deficit disorder. *Journal
of Consulting and Clinical Psychology, 65,* 749–757.

Power, T.J., Karustis, J.L., & Habboushe, D.F. (2001). *Homework success for children with ADHD: A family-school intervention program.* New York: Guilford
Press.

Rapport, M.D., & Denney, C.B. (2000). Attention deficit hyperactivity disorder
and methylphenidate: Assessment and prediction of clinical response. In
L.L. Greenhill & B.B. Osman (Eds.), *Ritalin: Theory and practice* (2nd ed.,
pp. 45–70). Larchmont, NY: Mary Ann Liebert.

Rapport, M.D., Scanlan, S.W., & Denney, C.B. (1999). Attention-
deficit/hyperactivity disorder and scholastic achievement: A model of dual
developmental pathways. *Journal of Child Psychology and Psychiatry, 40,*
1169–1183.

Reid, R., & Lienemann, T.O. (2006). *Strategy instruction for students with learning
disabilities: What works for special needs learners.* New York: Guilford.

Robin, A.L., & Foster, S.L. (1989). *Negotiating parent-adolescent conflict: A behavioral family systems approach.* New York: Guilford Press.

Rowe, K.J., & Rowe, K.S. (1992). The relationship between inattentiveness in
the classroom and reading achievement (Part B): An explanatory study.
Journal of the American Academy of Child and Adolescent Psychiatry, 31,
357–368.

Sawyer, M.G., Rey, J.M., Arney, F.M., Whitham, J.N., Clark, J.J., & Baghurst, P.A.
(2004). Use of health and school-based services in Australia by young people with attention-deficit/hyperactivity disorder. *Journal of the American
Academy of Child and Adolescent Psychiatry, 43,* 1355–1363.

Schnoes, C., Reid, R., Wagner, M., & Marder, C. (2006). ADHD among students
receiving special education services: A national survey. *Exceptional Children,
72,* 483–496.

Semrud-Clikeman, M., Biederman, J., Sprich-Buckminster, S., Lehman, B.K.,
Faraone, S.V., & Norman, D. (1992). Comorbidity between ADDH and
learning disability: A review and report in a clinically referred sample.
Journal of the American Academy of Child and Adolescent Psychiatry, 31,
439–448.

Shapiro, E.S. (2003). *Behavioral Observation of Students in Schools—BOSS*
[Computer software]. San Antonio, TX: Psychological Corporation.

Sheridan, S.M. (1995). *The Tough Kid Social Skills book.* Longmont, CO: Sopris-
West.

Sheridan, S.M., Dee, C.C., Morgan, J.C., McCormick, M.E., & Walker, D. (1996).
A multimethod intervention for social skills deficits in children with ADHD
and their parents. *School Psychology Review, 25,* 57–76.

Shinn, M.R. (Ed.). (1998). *Advanced applications of curriculum-based measurement.*
New York: Guilford Press.

Silver, L.B. (1990). Attention deficit-hyperactivity disorder: Is it a learning disability or a related disorder? *Journal of Learning Disabilities, 23,* 394–397.

Stroes, A., Alberts, E., & Van der Meere, J.J. (2003). Boys with ADHD in social
interaction with a nonfamiliar adult: An observational study. *Journal of the
American Academy of Child and Adolescent Psychiatry, 42,* 295–302.

Vile Junod, R.E., DuPaul, G.J., Jitendra, A.K., Volpe, R.J., & Cleary, K.S. (2006).
Classroom observations of students with and without ADHD: Differences
across types of engagement. *Journal of School Psychology, 44,* 87–104.

Volpe, R.J., DuPaul, G.J., DiPerna, J.C., Jitendra, A.K., Lutz, J.G., Tresco, K.E., et al. (2006). Attention-deficit/hyperactivity disorder and scholastic achievement: A model of mediation via academic enablers. *School Psychology Review, 35*, 47–61.

Walker, H.M., & McConnell, S.R. (1988). *Walker-McConnell Scale of Social Competence and School Adjustment*. Austin, TX: PRO-ED.

Walker, H.M., Severson, H.H., & Feil, E. G. (1995). *Early Screening Project (ESP): A proven child find success*. Longmont, CO: Sopris West.

Wechsler, D. (1992). *Wechsler Individual Achievement Test manual*. San Antonio, TX: Psychological Corporation.

Weyandt, L.L. (2007). *An ADHD primer* (2nd ed.). Mahwah, NJ: Lawrence Erlbaum Associates.

Woodcock, R., McGrew, K., & Mather, N. (2003). *Woodcock-Johnson Tests of Achievement* (3rd ed.). Chicago: Riverside Publishing Company.

CHAPTER 6

Treatment Strategies

Given that attention-deficit/hyperactivity disorder (ADHD) is a chronic disorder that impairs functioning across home, school, and community settings, treatment must be long term, implemented across settings, and directed at both symptoms and areas of impairment. The most commonly used and effective interventions for ADHD include psychotropic medication (primarily stimulants) and behavioral strategies implemented in home and school settings. The purpose of this chapter is to describe these psychotropic and psychosocial treatments. We also briefly identify other treatments that have been touted for this disorder but lack empirical support.

Psychotropic Medication

FDA-Approved Medications

The medications in this category have been approved by the U.S. Food and Drug Administration (FDA) for use in individuals with ADHD. The FDA approval means they have met at least the minimal standards to be evidence based. The standards include two studies completed at multiple centers that include a design where the children are assigned on a random basis for a period of time either to receive the medication or a placebo and appropriate measures are taken to determine the effects. Both the families and the researchers do not know who received the medication or placebo until the study is completed. These are referred to as *randomized controlled trials*. In addition, the children need to then be continued on the medication for at least 1 year to determine if the medication is continuing to provide benefit and not causing significant side effects. This design is referred to as an *open label safety-efficacy study*.

Stimulant Medications

Stimulant medication has been one of the mainstays of treating individuals with ADHD, going back to the 1950s and 1960s when the condition was characterized as minimal brain damage. In fact, amphetamine as a treatment for behavioral disorders dates back to 1937. In a hospital for children with behavioral disorders, Bradley (1937) observed and reported appreciable behavioral improvement when the children were given Benzedrine to treat their headaches that occurred secondarily to them receiving spinal taps required to perform pneumoencephlograms.

Despite Bradley's report, clinical use of stimulants did not start in earnest until 10 to 20 years later, initially with dextroamphetamine and subsequently with methylphenidate. These two medications went through extensive studies in the 1970s (Kavale, 1982) and 1980s (Greenhill, Halperin, & Abikoff, 1999) and continue to be the first line of medication treatment for ADHD. Because the early medications were of short duration lasting 4–5 hours, they required administration 2–4 times a day. Attempts to find medications that could last longer on a single dose led initially to the development of a wax matrix methylphenidate compound (Ritalin SR) and a dextroamphetamine spansule (Dexedrine Spansules) (Pelham et al., 1990). However, the initial long-acting formulations were limited in expanding the duration of effects, likely because they did not take into consideration the need for the more rapid immediate rise in blood levels occurring with the immediate release and the need for a continued rise in blood levels to sustain the effects (Swanson et al., 1999). Other alternative medications such as pemoline or tricyclic antidepressants were also found to be efficacious, but they had more significant side effects or a narrower margin of safety (caused more serious side effects when the dose exceeded recommended levels).

The stimulant medications (dextroamphetamine, mixed amphetamine salts, and methylphenidate) are the most studied psychotropic medications. There have been numerous studies of these medications showing consistent results (King et al., 2006). Most researchers have studied the effects of methylphenidate on elementary school age children (Brown et al., 2005). In the studies on mostly elementary school age children, with appropriate titration, approximately 70% responded to the first stimulant medication with which they were treated. When those children who did not respond were systematically tried on a second stimulant medication in the same manner, a total of approximately 80%–90% responded (Jensen, Hinshaw, Swanson, et al., 2001). There are far fewer studies in adolescents and adults, but the response rates have been similar to those achieved in children (Spencer et al., 2005; Wolraich et al., 2005).

Although dextroamphetamine is approved for use in children as young as 3 years of age and methylphenidate is only approved for children 6 years and older, the decisions reflect circumstances of the medication approval process at the time they were approved rather than clear differences in scientific evidence. In studies done since FDA approval, in preschool-age children, the majority of the studies have examined methylphenidate (Kollins & Greenhill, 2006). The largest and most recent study was a multisite study that found methylphenidate to be safe and effective in 4- to 5-year-old children with ADHD (Greenhill et al., 2006). However, the researchers found these younger children to have slower metabolic rates so that lower doses and longer durations per dose are required. In addition, side effects were seen more frequently. As seen in older children, some degree of growth suppression was observed. The expected growth potential of the child and the family's concern about their child's height are important to consider when deciding to start treatment, and it is critical to closely monitor height. It may also be more difficult to establish the diagnosis in preschool children and because of the theoretical concern about starting when the central nervous system is in an earlier stage of development, it is best to use the cautious approach employed in the multisite study (Gleason et al., 2007). They first asked families to participate in a behavior-based parent training program for 14 weeks and only started medication on those children whose behavior was not significantly improved by the parenting program. For one third of the families enrolled, the behavioral intervention was sufficient to improve their child's behavior (Greenhill et al., 2006). Some of these children may subsequently require medication, but the intervention was able to delay its introduction to an older age where the risks and benefits are better defined.

In adolescents, the studies show similar effects to those seen in younger children. As with very small children, it may be somewhat more difficult to diagnose ADHD in adolescence if it has not been diagnosed at an earlier time (Shaw et al., 2006). In addition, adolescents may be less likely to accept medication therapy and therefore one should include them in the discussion about whether to start medication. The effects of medication therapy are similar in adolescents to those in children, as are the choices of medication and doses used. Adolescents with ADHD commonly have comorbid conditions, such as depression, anxiety disorders, bipolar disorder, and substance abuse disorder. In these situations, the choice of medication may be altered by the comorbid conditions (McGough et al., 2005; Murphy, Barkley, & Bush, 2002).

As noted earlier, with appropriate titration (i.e., starting at the lowest dose and then increasing at small intervals until the optimal dose with the least side effects is found), approximately 70% of children and adolescents will respond to whichever stimulant medication is chosen for initial therapy. Although children will vary in their response to the initial therapy both with regard to efficacy and adverse effects, it is not possible to predict the response for each individual child. Therefore, the choice of starting with either a methylphenidate or amphetamine product is primarily dependent on the personal preferences of the families and their clinicians. If the response to the initially chosen medication is not beneficial, it is useful to try the alternative group (i.e., methylphenidate vs. amphetamine). The clinical response to stimulants is not related to weight or any other identifiable characteristics, such as severity of the behavioral symptoms. Therefore, it is most useful to titrate children systematically, first starting at the lowest dose and titrating up until attaining a maximal effect or causing significant adverse effects. It is best to obtain parent and teacher ratings of ADHD symptoms at each dosage, and these ratings should be compared to behavior observed when the children are not receiving medication. If the maximal dose is attained without appreciable improvement in the core symptoms, then it is useful to try a medication from the alternative stimulant medication group in the same manner. In this way, a total of approximately 80%–90% of children will respond to one of the stimulants (Wigal et al., 1999).

The stimulant medications reduce the core symptoms of inattention, hyperactivity, and impulsivity. They also improve academic productivity, although they do not improve cognitive abilities or academic skills. Furthermore, in some children, stimulants will reduce oppositional, aggressive, impulsive, and delinquent behaviors. It is helpful to measure medications by determining their impact on the children's core symptoms. These symptoms are most likely to show a noticeable change in response to medication and are likely to be the cause of impairment in a child with ADHD.

Although the evidence for the short-term efficacy in addressing the core symptoms of stimulant medications is quite clear, the evidence for long-term efficacy is not as clear (Ingram, Hechtman, & Morgenstern, 1999). Results from the National Institute of Mental Health's Multimodal Treatment Study of Children with ADHD support strong efficacy for 14 months when administered in a careful and systematic fashion (Jensen, Hinshaw, Swanson, et al., 2001). However, these children were followed for an additional 7 years (Molina et al., 2009) when they were no longer receiving the same intensive systematic care, and some no longer remained on medication. Some continued on medication and were continuing to improve, some remained improved despite stopping their medication, and in some the initial improvement on medication was not sustained even if they remained on medication. Longer-term studies in preschoolers and adolescents are lacking.

The three medications—dextroamphetamine, methylphenidate, and mixed amphetamine salts (75% dextroamphetamine and 25% levoamphetamine, having similar effects to dextroamphetamine)—have similar effects, side effects, and safety patterns. However, there are differences in plasma curves and duration of action, dependent on the delivery systems of the medications. In addition, while methylphenidate may lower the seizure threshold and dextroamphetamine and mixed amphetamine salts do not, all these medications have been used to treat children with ADHD and seizure disorders with no recurrence of seizures, as long as the seizure disorder is adequately controlled. Even in individuals with other comorbid conditions, such as anxiety or mood disorders, it is generally preferable to first treat the ADHD with stimulant medications because the mood or anxiety symptoms may diminish significantly if the stress caused by the ADHD is reduced. In those instances where the mood or anxiety disorder is causing a great deal of symptoms, however, it may be preferable to initiate therapy with a medication or behavioral interventions for these symptoms prior to starting a stimulant medication.

There are several misconceptions about stimulant medications. The effects of the medications are not paradoxical; that is, the reason individuals with ADHD seem calmer and more focused when taking a stimulant medication is due to the fact that the medication is ameliorating the underlying core ADHD symptoms. Stimulant medications act as dopamine and norepinephrine agonists or enhancers that block their reuptake, making them more available primarily in the caudate nucleus and prefrontal cortex. It is generally accepted that the pathophysiological basis of ADHD is a relative deficiency of dopamine and norepinephrine in those areas of the brain. Secondly, a response to medication cannot be used as a diagnostic test for ADHD. Because stimulants can improve performance in a variety of areas, individuals without ADHD may also see improved performance if they take the medications. Conversely, if an individual does not respond to a stimulant, it does not rule out the diagnosis of ADHD, because a minority of those individuals with ADHD will not respond to medication. Children, adolescents, and adults who are treated for ADHD usually do not find stimulant medication pleasurable and do not commonly abuse them. In individuals who do abuse stimulant medication, they usually have to take the medications intranasally or intravenously to obtain the euphoric feeling they seek. Abusers also usually require doses that are 10–100 times the dosage recommended for treating individuals with ADHD (Volkow & Swanson, 2003).

Table 6.1 lists the various formulations of the stimulant medications.

Methylphenidate   Methylphenidate is a racemic compound, meaning that it contains both the levo (left) and dextro (right) isomers of methylphenidate. The levo isomer is rapidly metabolized and essentially inactive. Short-acting methylphenidate has a half-life of 2–3 hours and a duration of action of approximately 4 hours. Within the past several years, there has been an increase in the number of delivery systems available to administer methylphenidate. The new delivery systems help to extend the duration of action of the medication. The purpose of extending the duration is to reduce the frequency of doses required for treatment and, particularly, to avoid having to administer the medications at school. The oldest compound is sustained-release methylphenidate. The extension of duration of action of this delivery system has been less than initially expected. It generally lasts approximately 5 hours. A newly improved system that utilizes microbead technology (intermediate-release methylphenidate) has extended the duration to 8 hours (equivalent to twice-daily dosing of regular methylphenidate) by using a mixture of immediate- and delayed-release beads. The medications primarily vary in the ratio of immediate- and delayed-release beads: a 50/50 ratio of immediate- to extended-release beads in Ritalin LA and a 30/70 ratio in Metadate CD. Therefore, children requiring a larger immediate response will respond better to Ritalin LA, whereas those requiring more in the afternoon will respond better to Metadate CD. The extended-release formulation of dexmethylphenidate (Focalin XR) is also a 50/50 mixture of immediate- and extended-release beads but appears to have a more extended release time, up to in some cases 12 hours. The system that uses an osmotic pump (extended-release OROS methylphenidate; Concerta) has the greatest extended duration of action of 10–12 hours. The capsule does not dissolve in the gastrointestinal system, so it is important to check if children have any constrictors or a narrowing in the gastrointestinal tract before prescribing this medication. A methylphenidate skin patch (Daytrana) also is able to provide

Table 6.1. Food and Drug Administration approved medications

	Brand names	Starting dose	Maximum dose	Daily frequency	How supplied
Stimulant medications					
Mixed amphetamine salts	Adderall	2.5–5 mg/day	40 mg/day	2–3 times/day	5 mg, 7.5 mg, 10 mg, 12.5 mg, 15 mg, 20 mg, and 30 mg tablets
	Adderall XR	10 mg/day	40 mg/day	1 time/day	5 mg, 10 mg, 15 mg, 20 mg, 25 mg, and 30 mg capsules
Dextroamphetamine	Dexedrine/Dextrostat	2.5 mg/day	40 mg/day	2–3 times/day	5 mg and (Dextrostat only) 10 mg tablets
	Dexedrine Spasules	5 mg/day	40 mg/day	1 time/day	5 mg, 10 mg, and 15 mg capsules
Lisdexamfetamine	Vyvanse	30 mg/day	70 mg/day	1 time/day	30 mg, 40 mg, 50 mg, 60 mg, and 70 mg capsules
Methylphenidate	Methylin	5 mg/day	60 mg/day	2–3 times/day	5 mg, 10 mg, and 20 mg tablets
	Ritalin	5 mg/day	60 mg/day	2–3 times/day	5 mg, 10 mg, and 20 mg tablets
	Ritalin SR	20 mg/day	60 mg/day	1–2 times/day	20 mg capsules
	Ritalin LA	20 mg/day	60 mg/day	1 time/day	20 mg, 30 mg, and 40 mg capsules
	Metadate CD	20 mg/day	60 mg/day	1 time/day	10 mg, 20 mg, 30 mg, 40 mg, 50 mg, and 60 mg capsules

(continued)

Table 6.1. (continued)

	Brand names	Starting dose	Maximum dose	Daily frequency	How supplied
	Concerta	18 mg/day	72 mg/day	1 time/day	18 mg, 36 mg, and 54 mg capsules
	Daytrana	10 mg/day	30 mg/day	apply for 9 hours	10 mg, 15 mg, 20 mg, and 30 mg patches
Dexmethylphenidate	Focalin	2.5 mg/day	30–40 mg/day	2 times/day	2.5 mg, 5 mg, and 10 mg tablets
	Focalin XR	5 mg/day	30–40 mg/day	1 time/day	5 mg, 10 mg, 15 mg, and 20 mg capsules
Selective norepinephrine reuptake inhibitors					
Atomoxetine	Strattera	0.5 mg/kg/day	1.4 mg/kg/day	1–2 times/day	10 mg, 18 mg, 25 mg, 40 mg, 60 mg, 80 mg, and 100 mg capsules
Alpha 2A adrenergic agonist					
Guanfacine	Intuniv	1 mg/day	4 mg/day	1 time/day	1 mg, 2 mg, 3 mg, and 4 mg tablets

extended effects for up to 12 hours. The duration can be tailored to the child's needs by removing the patch sooner than the 9 hours recommended for providing a 12-hour duration. It is important to note that the actual duration of action for any of these medications will vary from child to child (Greenhill et al., 1999).

The most common adverse side effects of methylphenidate are decreased appetite, sleep disturbance, and headache. The decreased appetite will frequently diminish after several months. If the child's weight is affected, use of calorie-enriched food may be helpful to reduce this side effect. It is important to determine the child's current and past history of sleep and headaches. Sleep problems are frequently present in children with ADHD independent of their treatments. When children are overly sensitive to the medication or they are given too high a dose, they may develop psychotic symptoms or become overfocused. These side effects can sometimes be resolved with lowering the dose. Overfocusing usually manifests by the child becoming listless—or what parents refer to "as appearing like a zombie." Methylphenidate can also have an effect on tics, chronic tic disorders, and Tourette syndrome. However, this effect is sometimes difficult to determine because the usual course of tics and tic disorders is for the tics to wax and wane. If children have tics and require methylphenidate, approximately one third will have an increase in the tics, approximately one third will have a decrease in the tics, and approximately one third will see no effect on their tics (Tourette's Syndrome Study Group, 2002).

Because the response of stimulant medication is so variable from child to child, doses related to the size of the child (mg/kg) are not as relevant as they are in children for other medications. The most appropriate process is to start at the lowest dose (5 mg/dose for methylphenidate or 2.5 mg/dose in children under 5 years of age) and gradually increase the dose until the optimal dose is achieved with the least side effects, up to the maximum dose of 60 mg/day (or 20 mg/dose of immediate-release formulations). The immediate-release methylphenidate preparations can be given two or three times daily based on the child's need for symptomatic relief and the family's preferences. Intermediate- and extended-release preparations are generally given once a day, which makes administration easier for parents and children. However, if a more extended time is required, the 8-hour preparations require an additional immediate-release formulation to be given in the afternoon in order to cover the rest of the day. This treatment plan with a reduced afternoon dose can be used in situations where an extended-release preparation causes an increase in sleep difficulties. Some children only require coverage for 8 hours. For example, those children with the inattentive subtype that is primarily creating school dysfunction may get by with morning and noontime dosing or one dose of an 8-hour preparation, while children with the combined type are more likely to require three times daily dosing or a 12-hour extended-release preparation because they are dysfunctional at both school and home.

The new extended-release formulations all have some immediate-release components. For OROS methylphenidate (Concerta), the equivalent of 10 mg methylphenidate three times daily is 36 mg, with 8 mg of immediate release. For Ritalin LA or dexmethylphenidate (Focalin XR), the ratio of immediate to extended release is 50/50, so they are 20-mg capsules that are equivalent to 10 mg twice daily and have 10 mg immediate release. Metadate CD, with a 30/70 ratio, has 6 mg immediate release.

Although obtaining a complete blood count periodically is in the original instructions for the prescription of methylphenidate, it has not been found to be needed and no specific laboratory assessments are required. Because the blood levels of methylphenidate do not correlate well with behavioral changes, they are also of little clinical use. The American Heart Association has recently recommended screening for a history of cardiac disease and obtaining an electrocardiogram (EKG) because of very rare cases of sudden death found in postmarketing surveillance. However, it is not clear that individuals being treated with stimulant medications are at any increased risk over the population in general, as the rates of sudden cardiac death in children not taking stimulant medications are similar. Although episodes of sudden cardiac death are obviously devastating, they are extremely rare. Therefore, the cost and difficulty of obtaining EKGs and the effects of false positives are reasons why the recommendations of the American Heart Association are not supported by the American Academy of Pediatrics or the American Academy of Child and Adolescent Psychiatry. However, it is important to perform a careful family history for sudden cardiac death, early onset of myocardial infarctions, and congenital heart disease as these may suggest the possibility of increased risk for significant arrhythmias, premature atherosclerosis, or hypertrophic or other cardiomyopathies. A personal history for hypertension, heart disease, chest pain, palpitations, shortness of breath, syncope, or dizziness with exertion should be sought. In addition, a cardiac examination and monitoring of blood pressure and heart rate should be undertaken. Abnormal findings should be fully assessed and a referral to a pediatric cardiologist should be considered before starting a child with abnormal findings on any stimulant medications.

Amphetamines The profile of action and side effects for amphetamines is very similar to that of methylphenidate. Short-acting dextroamphetamine has a half-life of 3–4 hours and a duration of action of approximately 5 hours. Like methylphenidate, the most common adverse side effects are anorexia (appetite suppression), sleep disturbance, and headache. The side effects profiles between methylphenidate and amphetamines are essentially the same, with the exception of several minor differences. There is more appetite suppression with dextroamphetamine, and dextroamphetamine does not lower the seizure threshold. The decreased appetite will frequently diminish after several months, but if the child's weight is affected, use of calorie-enriched food may be helpful. It is important to determine the child's current and past history of sleep and headaches. As stated previously, sleep problems are frequently present in children with ADHD independent of their treatments. Like methylphenidate, children who are overly sensitive or receive too high a dose may develop psychotic symptoms or become overfocused. These side effects can sometimes be resolved with lowering the dose. Overfocusing usually manifests by the child becoming listless—what parents refer to as "appearing like a zombie." The same challenges in determining the impact of methylphenidate on tics is true for amphetamines.

Like methylphenidate, because the response of stimulant medication is so variable from child to child, doses related to the size of the child (mg/kg) are not as relevant as they are in children for other medications. The most appropriate process is to start at the lowest dose (5 mg/dose or 2.5 mg/dose in children under 5 years of age) and gradually increase the dose until the optimal dose is achieved with the least side effects with the maximum dose being 40 mg/day. The dextroamphetamine can be given two or three times a day based on the child's need for symptomatic relief and the family's preferences. It has a slightly longer duration of action than methylphenidate. Like methylphenidate, no laboratory tests need to be monitored and blood levels are not of clinical utility, and the same is true for the issue of obtaining EKGs (Greenhill et al., 1999).

Mixed Amphetamine Salts Mixed amphetamine salts (Adderall) are mixtures of 75% dextroamphetamine and 25% levoamphetamine. Adderall appears to have a longer duration of action than methylphenidate, but it has never been assessed compared to dextroamphetamine, so it is unknown if it is any different in its treatment or side effects profile. The extended-release formulation (Adderall XR) using the extended bead technology (50% immediate release and 50% delayed release) has a longer and probably more effective duration of action, generally considered to be 10–12 hours in duration (Faraone, 2007).

   Lisdexamfetamine   Lisdexamfetamine (Vyvanse) is a prodrug that converts to dextroamphetamine in the bloodstream due to the action of a peptidase in red blood cells, which cleaves the lysine molecule. As a prodrug, it does not become active as an amphetamine until after it is ingested. This characteristic lowers the ability for it to be diverted and abused via intranasal or intravenous routes. However, at this point it has similar restrictions for use (Class II) as other stimulant medications. The metabolic process also results in a longer duration of action, usually only requiring a once-daily administration to provide 10- to 12-hour coverage. A recent study demonstrated efficacy at 13 hours after intake (Najib, 2009).

Nonstimulant Medications

There has been an interest in finding alternative medications to stimulants for treating ADHD for those children who do not respond to either class of stimulants or have severe or intolerable side effects. In addition, alternatives have been sought in order to have medications that don't have the Class II restrictions and can be used for individuals with ADHD and substance abuse issues or with individuals when there is concern that family members with substance abuse problems could divert their medications.

   Atomoxetine (Strattera)   Atomoxetine is a selective norepinephrine reuptake inhibitor. Its efficacy in treating children with ADHD is based on over 30 randomized control studies and approval by the FDA for treating ADHD in children, adolescents, and adults. Atomoxetine has a half-life of 4–19 hours. It is typically prescribed once per day but can also be given in two divided doses. The common adverse side effects of atomoxetine include appetite suppression, gastrointestinal upset, and somnolence. Rarely, hepatotoxicity can occur and rare reports of increased suicidal thoughts with no suicidal attempts found in reanalysis of the children who participated in the initial studies have prompted the FDA to issue a warning to monitor for this issue. Atomoxetine is metabolized through the cytochrome P450, 2D6. There are some children who are slow metabolizers, although most are extensive metabolizers. The clinical relevance of identifying slower metabolizers is not yet clear.

   Atomoxetine does not have abuse potential and is therefore not a Class II medication. Atomoxetine does not provide the rapid behavioral changes seen with stimulant medication, so the improvements may not be as noticeable, particularly to children and families who have used stimulant medications prior to a trial with atomoxetine. The slower changes emphasize the importance of monitoring the core symptoms through interview or rating scales to assess the effect of the medication during titration because the changes are likely to be more subtle. Although the effects documented in the controlled trials were for the daytime period, there is a suggestion that the medication effects may last more than 10 hours (Vaughan, Fegert, & Kratochvil, 2009).

Alpha-Adrenergic Agents   The other newly approved medication is an extended formulation of an alpha 2 agonist, guanfacine (Intuniv). Prior to the recent approval, the alpha-adrenergic medications used to treat patients with ADHD were clonidine (Catapres) and guanfacine (Tenex). While they were approved as antihypertensive agents, as alpha-noradrenergic agonists they also affect the central nervous system. Until recently they were not approved by the FDA because of limited evidence and lack of interest by any pharmaceutical company to seek approval. Recent approval of the extended release formulation of guanfacine (Intuniv) was obtained based on two large multisite randomized controlled trial studies (Biederman, Melmed, Patel, McBurnett, Konow, et al., 2008; Sallee et al., 2009) and two long-term safety efficacy open label trials (Biederman, Melmed, Patel, McBurnett, Donahue, et al., 2008; Sallee, Lyne, Wigal, & Donahue, 2009). There has also been one smaller study in children with ADHD and tic disorders (Scahill et al., 2001). Guanfacine is slower in action than stimulants, with a half-life of 24–36 hours. The recommended daily dose is 1–4 mg/day for guanfacine. The side effects of guanfacine include sedation, fatigue, anorexia, dry mouth, and hypotension. The sedation for guanfacine is less than that for clonidine. Tapering the medication in decrements of no more than 1 mg every 3–7 days when discontinuing its use is recommended to decrease the chance for a rebound increase in blood pressure.

Non–FDA-Approved Medications That Have Been Used to Treat ADHD

The medications in this category have not been approved by the FDA for use in individuals with ADHD. These medications have not had sufficient evidence to demonstrate their efficacy, have more severe side effects, or have a narrow margin of safety. They are not recommended for use unless the stimulant medications atomoxetine and extended-release guanfacine have been tried first and proved to be ineffective or have resulted in significant side effects. In addition, behavioral interventions with better efficacy evidence should also have been tried before considering a secondary medication.

Alpha-Adrenergic Medications

The immediate-release alpha-adrenergic medications used to treat children with ADHD are clonidine (Catapres) and guanfacine (Tenex). Although they were approved as antihypertensive agents, they are alpha-noradrenergic agonists that affect the central nervous system. However, their evidence of efficacy in treating children with ADHD is limited to two studies. More recently, additional studies completed on a long-acting form of guanfacine has been approved by the FDA and was described previously. The alpha-adrenergic medications are slower in action than stimulants, with a half-life of 24–36 hours. The average daily dose is 0.5–4 mg/day. The adverse side effects of the alpha-adrenergic medications include sedation (more so with clonidine), fatigue, anorexia (appetite suppression), dry mouth, and hypotension. There have been several cases of sudden death in children treated with a combination of clonidine and methylphenidate, but it has not been confirmed that the deaths were due to the medications. It is also important to taper the medication slowly when discontinuing its use and to monitor the child's blood pressure closely when the child is on the medication. A common use of clonidine is as an aid to sleep, a common problem in individuals with ADHD (Palumbo et al., 2008; Posey & McDougle, 2007).

Tricyclic Antidepressants

The tricyclic antidepressants used to treat children with ADHD have generally been imipramine (Tofranil), desipramine (Norpramin), and nortriptyline (Pamelor). Their mechanism of action is to inhibit the reuptake of serotonin and norepinephrine, but they also have anticholinergic effects. Their efficacy in the treatment of ADHD has been supported by approximately 20 randomized control trial studies. The tricyclic antidepressant medications are long acting and take several days to achieve a therapeutic level. Their mean half-life is 28–36 hours and the average daily dose is 25–150 mg (1–5 mg/kg). The minor side effects of the tricyclic antidepressant medications include sedation, anticholinergic effects such as dry mouth, and anorexia (appetite suppression), but the most significant side effect is cardiac arrhythmia. Most of the arrhythmias have been related to overdoses because of the narrow margin of safety, but at least for desipramine there may have been a sudden death at a therapeutic level. When prescribing the tricyclic antidepressant medications, it is important to monitor EKGs at baseline and then at each major dose change until an optimal dose is achieved. Blood levels should also be monitored to maintain a level between 150–250 ng/ml (Banaschewski, Roessner, Dittmann, Santosh, & Rothenberger, 2004).

Bupropion

Bupropion (Wellbutrin) is an antidepressive medication whose mechanism of action is mostly unclear. It is a weak dopamine agonist and it decreases whole body norepinephrine, but neither of these effects appears to explain its clinical results. Its efficacy in treating children with ADHD is derived from one multisite study where it was significantly better than placebo, but not as potent as stimulant medications. Bupropion has a half-life of 8–24 hours and is prescribed two or three times per day. The adverse side effects of bupropion include agitation, reduction in the seizure threshold, anorexia, insomnia, and nausea/vomiting. The appropriate dose range for treating children with bupropion is 50–75 mg two or three times daily. It requires no laboratory monitoring (Conners et al., 1996).

Modafinil

Modafinil (Provigil) is a wakefulness-promoting agent approved to treat sleep disorders such as narcolepsy in adults. Three recent studies of modafinil have been completed on children with ADHD with a total of 638 children, which showed significant improvement compared to a placebo. However, it was not approved by the FDA for the treatment of ADHD due to the development of Stevens-Johnson syndrome presenting with a skin rash, a potentially serious drug reaction, in two of the children in the study. The half-life for modafinil is 15 hours in adults. The doses tested in the three controlled studies in children with ADHD were 340 mg for children under 30 kg and 425 mg for those at or over 30 kg in two of the studies. The third study used a variable titrated dose and had a mean dose of 361 mg. The dose was titrated at dose intervals of 85-mg increments at days 1, 3, 8, 15, and 22. The most common adverse side effects are insomnia, headaches, and decreased appetite (Biederman & Pliszka, 2008).

Medication Management

Because the response to a particular medication is highly idiosyncratic across individuals, it is important to employ a systematic process to determine the most efficacious medication and dose for a child. It is also important to prepare families for the fact that the process may take up to a month or two in order to determine what is the best treatment for their child. Because methylphenidate and amphetamines have similar properties, it is the personal preference of the children, their families, and the clinicians as to which medication to start first. It is best to start at the lowest dose, the equivalent of 2.5 mg of methylphenidate for preschool-age children and 5 mg for children and adults or 2.5 mg of an amphetamine compound for children and adults twice or three times a day. The doses can be increased every 3–7 days at 2.5 mg/dose or 5 mg/dose up to a 40 mg of amphetamine (60 mg of methylphenidate). If after reaching the highest dose in the first choice of stimulant medication group (methylphenidate or amphetamine) the child is not manifesting improvement or significant side effects occur, it is worthwhile to try a medication from the other group.

The best method to determine a child's initial response to the medication is to monitor the 18 core symptoms used to establish the diagnosis. Rating scales that are based on the *Diagnostic and Statistical Manual of Mental Disorders, Fourth Edition* (American Psychiatric Association, 1994) criteria such as the Vanderbilt Rating Scales (Wolraich, Feurer, Hannah, Pinnock, & Baumgaertel, 1998) or ADHD Rating Scale IV (DuPaul, Power, Anastopoulos, & Reid, 1998) can provide that information from parents and teachers. The clinician should try to achieve at least a 25%–35% decrease in symptoms, although with many children it is possible to achieve a 50%–70% reduction in the number and severity as scored on the 0–3 scale of the core symptoms. It is best when, if at all possible, information about the core symptoms comes from more than one source. In children, the sources usually consist of the parent and teacher because children are not accurate reporters of their own behaviors. However, adolescents are typically better able to offer self-assessments of efficacy and adverse effects, although they are no more accurate than younger children (Kramer et al., 2004; Romano, Tremblay, Vitaro, Zoccolillo, & Pagani, 2001; Smith, Pelham, Gnagy, Molina, & Evans, 2000).

During the titration phase, it is possible to conduct the monitoring through phone calls, faxes, e-mails, or web-based data systems. For more long-term monitoring, it is helpful to have monthly visits for the first 6 months. In addition to checking height, weight, and blood pressure, it is recommended to check with the child and parents about both beneficial effects and side effects in more detail. At these visits it is also a good time to review the target goals to determine if the changes in core symptoms are improving the function as defined by the goals. Subsequently, if the improvements remain stable, ongoing management visits can be spaced less frequently depending on the child's needs.

The length of time daily that requires coverage using stimulant medications is an important discussion to have with the family. Children with the inattentive type of ADHD who do not have much homework may be able to manage on 8 hours of coverage with weekend and summer holidays, particularly for families who desire to minimize the medication use as much as possible. Alternatively, children with the combined type are more likely to need 12 hours of coverage and require medication 7 days a week. Adolescents need to consider the times they are likely to be driving as important times to have medication coverage. College students may have more chaotic and varied days that become more difficult to arrange for broad coverage and may ask about using immediate release formulations at targeted times such as studying, taking examinations, or writing papers. Adolescents also have to be warned about preventing diversion of the medication and that if they are involved in that process, they can incur significant legal jeopardy.

Although atomoxetine also requires some titration, it is different than for the stimulant medications because the effects are not as rapid. The changes are likely to occur more gradually over a 2- to 4-week period and the changes may not be as noticeable. Use of parent and teacher rating scales to monitor core symptoms can help to objectify the changes. Extended release guanfacine is also slower in manifesting effects.

Many children stop taking their medications after several years. Although there are many children who improve in their abilities to compensate for their core symptoms and can manage to function without medication, there are many who continue to see benefits on treatment. The extent to which individuals will continue to follow a treatment regimen is dependent on how much they and their parents know about their condition, the benefits they perceive to be the results of the treatment, how bothersome the side effects are, and how the medication is administered.

Psychosocial Treatment

The most effective psychosocial treatments are those that involve behavior modification strategies implemented by parents and teachers in home and school settings, respectively (for review, see Pelham & Fabiano, 2008). Specifically, the use of positive reinforcement and mild punishment techniques has been associated with relatively large effects (i.e., effect size > .80) on symptom-related behaviors and associated impairments (Fabiano et al., 2009). In addition, group and individual interventions aimed at enhancing social behavior and peer relationships have been effective when implemented consistently in applied settings (Pelham & Fabiano, 2008).

Home-Based Behavioral Treatment

The development of ADHD involves a complex interaction between biological (genetic) and environmental factors (Nigg, 2006). Thus, the family environment certainly contributes to the genesis and maintenance of challenging behaviors such as noncompliance, anger control, and aggression. Many research studies have documented the effectiveness of behavioral parent training in ameliorating these difficulties, at least over the short term (see Pelham & Fabiano, 2008). Parent training involves providing parents with direct instruction in behavior modification techniques to reduce problem behaviors and enhance family interactions. Specifically, parents are trained to identify problem behaviors, describe these in objective terms, collect rudimentary assessment information, and implement strategies that involve anticipating and responding to behavior in a different manner. There are several published parent training programs that are designed for children with ADHD and related disruptive behavior disorders (e.g., Barkley, 1987; Cunningham, Bremner, & Secord-Gilbert, 1998; Webster-Stratton, 1996). Although parent training protocols may differ with regard to specific components (e.g., use of token reinforcement and punishment), there are several underlying principles and procedures that are common to all effective training programs.

An important component of all parent training programs is systematic instruction in the use of empirically supported behavioral strategies. These strategies include the modification of antecedent and consequent events, as well as direct changes to the target behavior. Antecedents or "triggers" are those environmental events that occur prior to a target behavior, while consequences or "responses" are environmental events that occur after a target behavior is emitted. Preventive strategies involve parents changing antecedent events prior to a behavior occurring. For example, if a child throws a tantrum when abruptly asked to make the transition from one activity to another (e.g., clean up toys and come to dinner table), then a preventive strategy might involve parents giving one or two warnings prior to the transition. Instructive strategies are directed at providing the child with a different and more appropriate way to accomplish a goal. For example, if it is determined that a child gets frustrated and becomes inattentive when doing a long homework assignment, then the child can be taught to request a break at several points during the homework period. Requesting a break is a more appropriate way to temporarily avoid frustration than is becoming distracted and inattentive.

Consequence-based strategies involve modifying consequent events in order to change a target behavior. Consequence-based strategies include those that are designed to increase a behavior referred to as positive reinforcement (e.g., parental praise, token reinforcement). Alternatively, strategies designed to decrease a specific behavior are referred to as punishment (e.g., time-out from positive reinforcement, response cost). All parent training programs emphasize the more frequent use of positive reinforcement relative to punishment. Furthermore, an effective home-based behavior modification plan will include all three components (preventive, instructive, and consequence-based). In fact, when all three components are included, this is often more time-efficient and cost-effective because the need for consequences are reduced (presumably due to the effects of preventive and instructive approaches).

A second important feature common to all parent training programs is the sequential exposure to behavior modification principles over an extended period of time. This sequential and spaced delivery of information increases the odds that parents will understand the rationale and specifics of each procedure and also will have the opportunity to practice prescribed strategies between sessions. Typically, parent education is delivered in 8 or more weekly or biweekly sessions conducted over 2 or more months. Parents are initially informed about ADHD and related behavior disorders in a developmental context. Then, antecedent-based preventive strategies are covered, followed by instructive strategies, and then consequent-based approaches. Positive reinforcement techniques are introduced prior to punishment because use of the former may preclude or reduce the need for the latter. Finally, one or two sessions are devoted to providing parents with strategies they can use to problem-solve on their own once treatment has ended. Many parent training programs also include one or more booster sessions that are held at a later point in order to help parents maintain the use of effective

Table 6.2. Example of parent training sequence of topics

Session	Topic
1	Overview of attention-deficit/hyperactivity disorder (ADHD) and related disorders
2	Overview of behavioral principles and common functions associated with challenging behaviors
3	Use of preventive strategies (e.g., effective commands)
4	Use of instructive strategies (e.g., direct instruction of alternate behaviors)
5	Paying attention to child behavior (consequence-based strategy)
6	Implementing a token reinforcement system (consequence-based strategy)
7	Use of time-out from positive reinforcement and response cost (consequence-based strategies)
8	Managing behavior in public places (e.g., restaurants, supermarket)
9	Anticipating future behavior problems
10	Booster session (2 months after Session 9)

techniques. Table 6.2 provides an example of topics covered in a typical parent training program.

A third important feature of parent training programs is that parents are provided with specific instructions in how to implement behavioral strategies and receive feedback from the therapist based on implementation results. Although programs differ with respect to the relative balance between didactic instruction, group discussion, and guided practice, all effective programs provide parents with specific step-by-step instructions on how interventions are to be implemented between training sessions. Homework (e.g., practice implementing prescribed technique) is assigned in one session and reviewed in the following session, thus offering therapists an opportunity to reinforce what parents are doing correctly and offer guidance in any necessary changes. It is this combination of specificity and feedback that is critical to the accurate implementation of strategies and encouragement of their consistent use over time.

A final critical feature of effective parent training programs is flexibility with respect to how content is delivered. Specifically, these programs can be delivered to individual sets of parents or in a group format. The individual format has the advantage of tailoring training content to a specific family's needs, while the group format is advantageous for providing parents with peer support. The decision as to individual vs. group parent training will be based on availability of resources, a specific family's needs, and therapist preferences. Importantly, efficacy of training does not appear to vary as a function of individual vs. group delivery.

Parent training in behavior modification typically is focused on the needs of preschool and elementary school age children. Very little research has been conducted with this approach for adolescents with ADHD. Robin (2006) has proposed a biobehavioral–family system approach to working with families of adolescents with this disorder. This treatment program includes elements that are effective with younger children, such as providing education about the disorder and implementing consistent behavioral procedures in the home. It differs from typical parent training in that 1) the adolescent (and entire family) participates, not just the parents; 2) a more abstract version of token reinforcement is used (i.e., behavioral contracting); 3) family communication patterns are modified to enhance clarity and consistency; and 4) families are taught problem-solving skills that can be used on an ongoing basis. Families are also provided with information about medication (if necessary) and homework is specifically targeted to enhance academic performance. This treatment program makes intuitive sense and includes components that are empirically supported; however, the efficacy of this program as a package needs to be established before widespread use can be recommended.

School-Based Behavioral Treatment

Behavioral interventions implemented in the school are similar to those discussed for the home setting and include preventive or proactive, instructive, and consequence-based or reactive strategies. As discussed in Chapter 8, interventions can be mediated by teachers, peers, parents, computers, or the students with ADHD themselves. Thus, a balanced and effective school-based treatment plan will include both proactive and reactive strategies that are implemented by two or more mediators (i.e., not just by the teacher). More details regarding specific school-based interventions are provided in Chapter 8. Many controlled studies have demonstrated the effectiveness of school-based behavioral strategies in increasing appropriate behavior, decreasing disruptive behavior, and, in some cases, enhancing academic and social functioning (for meta-analytic reviews, see DuPaul & Eckert, 1997; Fabiano et al., 2009).

Behavioral Peer Interventions

Children and adolescents with ADHD typically exhibit significant difficulties interacting with peers and may have difficulties making and keeping friends. The traditional approach to addressing these social interaction difficulties has been to teach children specific social skills (e.g., making eye contact and taking turns) that are assumed to be miss-ing from their behavioral repertoires. Group sessions are held for 60–90 minutes on a weekly basis, typically conducted in a therapy room or somewhere separate from the classroom or neighborhood. This social skills training approach has not been very successful, in large part because any skills learned in training tend not to generalize to settings outside of therapy sessions (Gresham, 2002; Pelham & Fabiano, 2008).

A more viable approach to enhancing peer relationships, referred to as *behavioral peer intervention*, involves treatment strategies that encourage children to use skills already in their repertoires by prompt-ing appropriate use and reinforcing generalization across settings (Pelham & Fabiano, 2008). Thus, rather than viewing children's peer relationship difficulties as arising from skills deficits, it is more accu-rate to focus on deficits in behavioral performance (Barkley, 2006). Stated differently, children need to learn when to and when not to engage in specific behaviors. This can only be accomplished by provid-ing treatment in situ rather than exclusively in the context of group training sessions conducted at a separate time and place from the behaviors of interest.

The effects of behavioral peer interventions have been most prominently evident in the context of summer treatment programs (STP) for children and adolescents with ADHD (Pelham & Fabiano, 2008). The STP involves participation in a full-day "summer camp" program for 5–8 weeks with children exposed to structured, contin-gency management programming throughout each day. The behav-ioral peer intervention component of STP includes brief social skills training sessions combined with intensive behavioral procedures to prompt and reinforce appropriate social behaviors during recre-ational activities. Specifically, adult facilitators coach (i.e., prompt) appropriate group play and provide both reinforcing (e.g., token rein-forcement or points) and punishing (e.g., time-out from positive rein-forcement) contingencies depending on behaviors exhibited by the children. In addition, parents provide home-based rewards for gains made in social behavior in the context of a daily report card system (see Chapter 8 for more details about daily report card systems). Team membership and sports skills also are taught as part of this comprehensive behavioral peer intervention program. The efficacy of this program has been demonstrated in numerous well-controlled studies primarily in the context of STP (e.g., Chronis et al., 2004). Given that this approach is much more time and resource intensive than traditional social skills training, it will be important for future research to document the efficacy and feasibility of behavioral peer interventions in school settings.

Other Psychosocial Treatments

Various nonbehavioral psychological treatments have been proposed as ADHD interventions, including cognitive therapy, play therapy, traditional "talk" therapy or psychotherapy, and family therapy (for review, see Barkley, 2006). Unfortunately, these approaches have little to no empirical support. The lack of efficacy for these treatments is not surprising given that they do not directly target mechanisms related to ADHD. Stated differently, ADHD does not appear to be caused by psychological trauma, internal psychic conflict, aberrant cognitions, or dysfunctional family interactions (Nigg, 2006). Furthermore, these psychosocial treatments are delivered far from the "point of performance" (Goldstein & Goldstein, 1998). The point of performance is the setting and time where the behavior of interest occurs. Given that ADHD may represent impaired delayed responding to the environment (Barkley, 1997), then it is critical that treatment is implemented as close to the point of performance as possible. If the behavior of interest is disruptive behavior that occurs in math class scheduled from 9:00 a.m. to 9:45 a.m. each day, then an intervention delivered at this point of performance will have a better chance of success than one delivered in the afternoon or in a different room. Thus, at the present time, effective psychosocial approaches to ADHD are those that are behaviorally based and are implemented by parents and teachers in home and school settings, respectively.

Combined Interventions

The two most efficacious treatments for ADHD are psychostimulant medication and behavioral interventions implemented in home and school settings. Research studies that have compared the relative effects of these two modalities typically indicate that stimulants produce the greatest effects on ADHD symptoms, while behavioral interventions are equal to or superior to stimulants in reducing defiant, aggressive behavior while enhancing social and academic functioning (Brown et al., 2008). To a large extent, this "horse race" approach to examining relative effects is counterproductive as it is rare for either treatment modality to be sufficient in addressing the myriad difficulties encountered by children with ADHD. Of greater clinical import are the many empirical studies that have documented the salutary effects of a combined treatment approach. In fact, the general consensus in the field is that the combination of stimulant medication and behavioral interventions is optimal for many children and adolescents with this disorder (e.g., American Academy of Pediatrics, 2001).

There are several potential advantages to a combined treatment strategy. First, although not consistently the case, some studies have shown that the combination of stimulants and behavioral interventions results in better outcomes than either treatment in isolation. This superior outcome is particularly prominent for children with comorbid disorders and/or for children from ethnically and socioeconomically diverse backgrounds (Arnold et al., 2003; Jensen, Hinshaw, Kraemer, et al., 2001). Second, a combined treatment protocol is more likely to address symptoms across time and settings. Because ADHD is a chronic disorder that affects functioning in a ubiquitous fashion, this is an important aspect of treatment. Third, there is evidence to suggest that combining treatments may allow use of lower dosages of each intervention. For example, Fabiano and colleagues (2007) found that the combination of low-intensity classroom behavioral intervention and low dosage of methylphenidate led to effects on disruptive behavior and academic productivity that were equivalent or superior to effects found for the high dosage of either treatment in isolation. Fourth, if lower dosages of each treatment can be used when these are combined, then the probability of adverse side effects is reduced and the overall treatment plan may be more palatable to parents and teachers.

Treatment Strategies without Empirical Support

Because ADHD is a chronic condition with no known cure, many treatments for this condition have been proposed over the years. Furthermore, because the two primary empirically supported approaches (i.e., psychostimulants and behavior modification) have limitations, parents and teachers are sometimes anxious to use alternative treatments that purportedly do not have the adverse side effects associated with medications and/or do not involve as much time and effort as the behavioral interventions. Examples of alternative treatments that have been proposed over the years include removing artificial food colorings and/or sugar from the diet, using St. John's wort or other herbal remedies, and electroencephalogram (EEG) biofeedback (Ingersoll & Goldstein, 1993). Although EEG biofeedback is beginning to receive some controlled empirical support (e.g., Gevensleben et al., 2009), these alternative treatment approaches have either not been researched or have only been examined in the context of uncontrolled or poorly controlled studies.

As we discuss in Chapter 11, there are a number of issues to consider when evaluating the support for any proposed treatment. First, the treatment should be supported by multiple empirical studies that control for threats to internal validity. Ideally, two or more investigative teams would have independently studied the treatment. Second, information about the treatment should come from a credible source such as a peer-reviewed scientific journal or a well-respected professional organization. Testimonials based on clinical experience do not qualify as credible sources no matter how strong the credentials of the individuals involved. Third, one should be wary of any treatments that are described as a cure for ADHD or are touted as effective for multiple disorders that are very different in etiology and presentation (e.g., autism, ADHD, schizophrenia). Finally, in order to be a viable alternative treatment for ADHD, any purported strategy should have demonstrated efficacy that is at least as strong as that found for ADHD psychotropic medications and behavioral interventions. Otherwise, there is no reason to abandon the most effective treatments for one that is less likely to succeed.

Conclusions

The most effective treatments for ADHD are psychotropic medication (primarily stimulants) and behavioral strategies implemented across home and school settings. It is clear from the empirical literature that the single most effective intervention for reducing ADHD symptoms is stimulant medication. In fact, the typical effect size for stimulant-induced change in ADHD symptoms is relatively large and exceeds 0.80 standard deviation units (Conners, 2002). Alternatively, even when medication results in clinically significant reduction in symptomatic behaviors, this does not regularly translate into improvements in academic achievement and peer relationships (e.g., MTA Cooperative Group, 1999, 2004). Behavioral interventions also lead to significant reductions in ADHD symptoms; however, the magnitude of effect is typically smaller than that found for stimulants. The impact of behavioral strategies is more pronounced on functional impairment, particularly in the social and academic domains with effect sizes in the moderate range (Fabiano et al., 2009).

Based on the available literature, we strongly recommend that behavioral interventions at home and school be implemented with all children and adolescents diagnosed with ADHD. There are minimal adverse side effects associated with this treatment, and there is potential for impacting both symptomatic behaviors as well as social and academic functioning. Medication should also be considered for most children with the disorder, particularly if symptoms are at least moderate in severity and/or prior psychosocial treatment has not been successful. Furthermore, there is growing evidence that the combination of stimulants and behavioral strategies is optimal for many children with the disorder as the effects of each treatment may complement each other. In fact, combining stimulants and behavioral techniques could be synergistic such that a lower dosage of each treatment may be possible when combined rather than implemented in isolation (e.g., Fabiano et al., 2007). Thus, combined treatment may not only be optimal for reducing symptoms and enhancing functioning but also may be associated with fewer adverse side effects and greater consumer acceptability due to the use of lower dosages of each treatment.

References

American Academy of Pediatrics, Subcommittee on Attention-Deficit/Hyperactivity Disorder and Committee on Quality Improvement. (2001). Clinical practice guideline: Treatment of the school-aged child with attention-deficit/hyperactivity disorder. *Pediatrics, 108,* 1033–1044.

American Psychiatric Association. (1994). *Diagnostic and statistical manual of mental disorders* (4th ed.). Washington, DC: Author.

Arnold, E., Elliott, M., Sachs, L., Kraemer, H.C., Abikoff, H.B., Conners, C.K., et al. (2003). Effects of ethnicity on treatment attendance, stimulant response/dose, and 14-month outcome in ADHD. *Journal of Consulting and Clinical Psychology, 71,* 713–727.

Banaschewski, T., Roessner, V., Dittmann, R.W., Santosh, P.J., & Rothenberger, A. (2004). Non-stimulant medications in the treatment of ADHD. *European Child and Adolescent Psychiatry, 13*(Suppl. 1), 102–116.

Barkley, R.A. (1987). *Defiant children: A clinician's manual for parent training.* New York: Guilford Press.

Barkley, R.A. (1997). *ADHD and the nature of self-control.* New York: Guilford Press.

Barkley, R.A. (Ed.). (2006). *Attention-deficit/hyperactivity disorder: A handbook for diagnosis and treatment* (3rd ed.). New York: Guilford Press.

Biederman, J., Melmed, R.D., Patel, A., McBurnett, K., Donahue, J., & Lyne, A. (2008). Long-term, open-label extension study of guanfacine extended release in children and adolescents with ADHD. *CNS Spectrums, 13*(12), 1047–1055.

Biederman, J., Melmed, R.D., Patel, A., McBurnett, K., Konow, J., Lyne, A., et al. (2008). A randomized, double-blind, placebo-controlled study of guanfacine extended release in children and adolescents with attention-deficit/hyperactivity disorder. *Pediatrics, 121,* e73–e84.

Biederman, J., & Pliszka, S.R. (2008). Modafinil improves symptoms of attention-deficit/hyperactivity disorder across subtypes in children and adolescents. *Journal of Pediatrics, 152,* 394–399.

Bradley, C. (1937). The behavior of children receiving benzedrine. *American Journal of Psychiatry, 94,* 577–585.

Brown, R., Amler, R.W., Freeman, W.S., Perrin, J.M., Stein, M.T., Feldman, H.M., et al. (2005). Treatment of attention-deficit/hyperactivity disorder: Overview of the evidence. *Pediatrics, 115,* e749–e756.

Brown, R.T., Antonuccio, D., DuPaul, G.J., Fristad, M., King, C.A., Leslie, L.K., et al. (2008). *Childhood mental health disorders: Evidence base and contextual factors for psychosocial, psychopharmacological, and combined interventions.* Washington, DC: American Psychological Association.

Chronis, A.M., Fabiano, G.A., Gnagy, E.M., Onyango, A.N., Pelham, W.E., Williams, A., et al. (2004). An evaluation of the Summer Treatment Program for children with attention-deficit/hyperactivity disorder using a treatment withdrawal design. *Behavior Therapy, 35,* 561–585.

Conners, C.K. (2002). Forty years of methylphenidate treatment in attention-deficit/hyperactivity disorder. *Journal of Attention Disorders, 6,* 17–30.

Conners, C., Casat, C., Gualtieri, C.T., Weller, E., Reader, M., Reiss, A., et al. (1996). Bupropion hydrochloride in attention deficit disorder with hyperactivity. *Journal of the American Academy of Child and Adolescent Psychiatry, 35,* 1314–1321.

Cunningham, C.E., Bremner, R.B., & Secord-Gilbert, M. (1998). *COPE, the Community Parent Education Program: A school based family systems oriented workshop for parents of children with disruptive behavior disorders (Leader's manual).* Hamilton, Ontario, Canada: COPE Works.

DuPaul, G.J., Power, T.J., Anastopoulos, A.D., & Reid, R (1998). *ADHD Rating Scale IV: Checklist, norms, and clinical interpretation.* New York: Guilford Press.

DuPaul, G.J., & Eckert, T.L. (1997). The effects of school-based interventions for attention deficit hyperactivity disorder: A meta-analysis. *School Psychology Review, 26,* 5–27.

Fabiano, G.A., Pelham, W.E., Jr., Coles, E.K., Gnagy, E.M., Chronis-Tuscano, A., & O'Connor, B.C. (2009). Meta-analysis of behavioral treatments for attention-deficit/hyperactivity disorder. *Clinical Psychology Review, 29,* 129–140.

Fabiano, G.A., Pelham, W.E., Jr., Gnagy, E.M., Burrows-MacLean, L., Coles, E.K., Chacko, A., et al. (2007). The single and combined effects of multiple intensities of behavior modification and methylphenidate for children with attention deficit hyperactivity disorder in a classroom setting. *School Psychology Review, 36,* 195–216.

Faraone, S. (2007). Stimulant therapy in the management of ADHD: Mixed amphetamine salts (extended release). *Expert Opinion on Pharmacotherapy, 8,* 2127–2134.

Gevensleben, H., Holl, B., Albrecht, B., Vogel, C., Schlamp, D., Kratz, O., et al. (2009). Is neurofeedback an efficacious treatment for ADHD? A randomized controlled clinical trial. *Journal of Child Psychology and Psychiatry, 50,* 780–789.

Gleason, M.M., Egger, H.L., Emslie, G.J., Greenhill, L.L., Kowatch, R.A., Lieberman, A.F., et al. (2007). Psychopharmacological treatment for very young children: Contexts and guidelines. *Journal of the American Academy of Child and Adolescent Psychiatry, 46,* 1532–1572.

Goldstein, S., & Goldstein, M. (1998). *Managing attention deficit hyperactivity disorder in children: A guide for practitioners* (2nd ed.). New York: Wiley.

Greenhill, L.L., Halperin, J.M., & Abikoff, H.B. (1999). Stimulant medications. *Journal of the American Academy of Adolescent Psychiatry, 38,* 503–512.

Greenhill, L., Kollins, S., Abikoff, H., McCracken, J., Riddle, M., Swanson, J., et al. (2006). Efficacy and safety of immediate-release methylphenidate treatment for preschoolers with ADHD. *Journal of the American Academy of Child and Adolescent Psychiatry, 45,* 1284–1293.

Gresham, F.M. (2002). Teaching social skills to high-risk children and youth: Preventive and remedial strategies. In M.R. Shinn, H.M. Walker, & G. Stoner (Eds.), *Interventions for academic and behavior problems: II. Preventive and remedial approaches* (2nd ed., pp. 403–432). Washington, DC: National Association of School Psychologists.

Ingersoll, B., & Goldstein, S. (1993). *Attention deficit disorder and learning disabilities: Realities, myths, and controversial treatments.* New York: Doubleday.

Ingram, S., Hechtman, L., & Morgenstern, G. (1999). Outcome issues in ADHD: Adolescent and adult long-term outcome. *Mental Retardation and Developmental Disabilities Research Reviews, 5,* 243–250.

Jensen, P.S., Hinshaw, S.P., Kraemer, H.C., Lenora, N., Newcorn, J.H., Abikoff, H.B., et al. (2001). ADHD comorbidity findings from the MTA study: Comparing comorbid subgroups. *Journal of the American Academy of Child and Adolescent Psychiatry, 40,* 147–158.

Jensen, P.S., Hinshaw, S.P., Swanson, J.M., Greenhill, L.L., Conners, C.K., Arnold, L.E., et al. (2001). Findings from the NIMH multimodal treatment study of ADHD (MTA): Implications and applications for primary care providers. *Journal of Developmental and Behavioral Pediatrics, 22,* 60–73.

Kavale, K. (1982). The efficacy of stimulant drug treatment for hyperactivity: A meta-analysis. *Journal of Learning Disabilities 15,* 280–289.

King, S., Griffin, S., Hodges, Z., Weatherly, H., Asseburg, C., Richardson, G., et al. (2006). A systematic review and economic model of the effectiveness and cost-effectiveness of methylphenidate, dexamfetamine and atomoxetine for the treatment of attention deficit hyperactivity disorder in children and adolescents. *Health Technology Assessment (Winchester, England), 10,* iii–iv, xiii–146.

Kollins, S.H., & Greenhill, L.L. (2006). Evidence base for the use of stimulant medication in preschool children with ADHD. *Infant and Young Children, 19,* 132–141.

Kramer, T.L., Phillips, S.D., Hargis, M.B., Miller, T.L., Burns, B.J., & Robbins, J.M. (2004). Disagreement between parent and adolescent reports of functional impairment. *Journal of Child Psychology and Psychiatry, 45,* 248–259.

McGough, J., Smalley, S.L., McCracken, J.T., Yang, M., Del'Homme, M., Lynn, D.E., et al. (2005). Psychiatric comorbidity in adult attention deficit hyperactivity disorder: Findings from multiplex families. *American Journal of Psychiatry, 162,* 1621–1627.

Molina, B., Hinshaw, S.P., Swanson, J.M., Arnold, L.E., Vitiello, B., Jensen, P.S., et al. (2009). The MTA at 8 years: Prospective follow-up of children treated for combined type ADHD in the multisite study. *Journal of the American Academy of Child and Adolescent Psychiatry, 48,* 484–500.

MTA Cooperative Group. (1999). A 14-month randomized clinical trial of treatment strategies for attention-deficit/hyperactivity disorder. *Archives of General Psychiatry, 56,* 1073–1086.

MTA Cooperative Group. (2004). National Institute of Mental Health multimodal treatment study of ADHD follow-up: 24-month outcomes of treatment strategies for attention-deficit/hyperactivity disorder. *Pediatrics, 113,* 754–761.

Murphy, K., Barkley, R.A., Bush, T. (2002). Young adults with attention deficit hyperactivity disorder: Subtype differences in comorbidity, educational and clinical history. *Journal of Nervous and Mental Disease, 190,* 147–157.

Najib, J. (2009). The efficacy and safety profile of lisdexamfetamine dimesylate, a prodrug of d-amphetamine, for the treatment of attention-deficit/hyperactivity disorder in children and adults. *Clinical Therapeutics, 31*, 142–176.

Nigg, J.T. (2006). *What causes ADHD?* New York: Guilford Press.

Palumbo, D., Sallee, F.R., Pelham, W.E., Jr., Bukstein, O.G., Daviss, W.B., & McDermott, M.P. (2008). Clonidine for attention-deficit/hyperactivity disorder: I. Efficacy and tolerability outcomes. *Journal of the American Academy of Child and Adolescent Psychiatry, 47*, 180–188.

Pelham, W.E., Jr., & Fabiano, G.A. (2008). Evidence-based psychosocial treatments for attention-deficit/hyperactivity disorder. *Journal of Clinical Child and Adolescent Psychology, 37*, 184–214.

Pelham, W., Greenslade, K.E., Vodde-Hamilton, M., Murphy, D.A., Greenstein, J.J., Gnagy, E.M., et al. (1990). Relative efficacy of long-acting stimulants on children with attention deficit hyperactivity disorder: A comparison of standard methylphenidate, sustained-release methylphenidate, sustained release dextroamphetamine, and pemoline. *Pediatrics, 86*, 226–236.

Posey, D., & McDougle, C.J. (2007). Guanfacine and guanfacine extended release: Treatment for ADHD and related disorders. *CNS Drug Reviews, 13*, 465–474.

Robin, A.L. (2006). Training families with adolescents with ADHD. In R.A. Barkley (Ed.), *Attention-deficit/hyperactivity disorder: A handbook for diagnosis and treatment* (3rd ed., pp. 499–546). New York: Guilford Press.

Romano, E., Tremblay, R.E., Vitaro, F., Zoccolillo, M., & Pagani, L. (2001). Prevalence of psychiatric diagnoses and the role of perceived impairment: Findings from an adolescent community sample. *Journal of Child Psychology and Psychiatry, 42*, 451–462.

Sallee, F.R., Lyne, A., Wigal, T., & Donahue, J. (2009). Long-term safety and efficacy of guanfacine extended release in children and adolescents with attention-deficit/hyperactivity disorder. *Journal of Child and Adolescent Psychopharmacology, 19*(3), 215–226.

Sallee, F.R., Mcgough, J., Wigal, T., Donahue, J., Lyne, A., & Biederman, J. (2009). Guanfacine extended release in children and adolescents with attention deficit hyperactivity disorder: A placebo-controlled trial. *Journal of the American Academy of Child and Adolescent Psychiatry, 48*, 155–165.

Scahill, L., Chappell, P.B., Kim, Y.S., Schultz, R.T., Katsovich, L., Shepherd, E., et al. (2001). A placebo-controlled study of guanfacine in the treatment of children with tic disorders and attention deficit hyperactivity disorder. *American Journal of Psychiatry, 158*(7), 1067–1074.

Shaw, P., Greenstein, D., Lerch, J., Clasen, L., Lenroot, R., Gogtay, N., et al. (2006). Intellectual ability and cortical development in children and adolescents. *Nature, 440*, 676–679.

Smith, B., Pelham, W.E., Jr., Gnagy, E., Molina, B., & Evans, S. (2000). The reliability, validity, and unique contributions of self-report by adolescents receiving treatment for attention-deficit/hyperactivity disorder. *Journal of Consulting and Clinical Psychology, 68*, 489–499.

Spencer, T., Biederman, J., Wilens, T., Doyle, R., Surman, C., Prince, J., et al. (2005). A large, double blind, randomized clinical trial of methylphenidate in the treatment of adults with attention deficit/hyperactive disorder. *Biological Psychiatry, 57*, 456–463.

Swanson, J.M., Gupta, S., Guinta, D., Flynn, D., Agler, D., Lerner, M., et al. (1999). Acute tolerance to methylphenidate in the treatment of attention deficit hyperactivity disorder in children. *Clinical Pharmacology and Therapeutics, 66,* 295–305.

Tourette's Syndrome Study Group. (2002). Treatment of ADHD in children with tics: A randomized controlled trial. *Neurology, 58,* 527–536.

Vaughan, B., Fegert, J., & Kratochvil, C.J. (2009). Update on atomoxetine in the treatment of attention-deficit/hyperactivity disorder. *Expert Opinion on Pharmacotherapy, 10,* 669–676.

Volkow, N.D., & Swanson, J.M. (2003). Variables that affect the clinical use and abuse of methylphenidate in the treatment of ADHD. *American Journal of Psychiatry, 160,* 1909–1918.

Webster-Stratton, C. (1996). *The Parents and Children Series: A comprehensive course divided into four programs.* Seattle, WA: Author.

Wigal, T., Swanson, J.M., Regino, R., Lerner, M.A., Soliman, I., Steinhoff, K., et al. (1999). Stimulant medications for the treatment of ADHD: Efficacy and limitations. *Mental Retardation and Developmental Disabilities Research Reviews, 5,* 215–224.

Wolraich, M.L., Wibbelsman, C.J., Brown, T.E., Evans, S.W., Gotlieb, E.M., Knight, J.R., et al. (2005). Attention deficit hyperactivity disorder in adolescents: A review of the diagnosis, treatment and clinical implications. *Pediatrics, 115,* 1734–1746.

Wolraich, M.L., Feurer, I., Hannah, J.N., Pinnock, T.Y., & Baumgaertel, A. (1998). Obtaining systematic teacher report of disruptive behavior disorders utilizing DSM-IV. *Journal of Abnormal Child Psychology, 26,* 141–152.

CHAPTER 7

The Family's Role

Family functioning is critically important in understanding attention-deficit/hyperactivity disorder (ADHD) because familial factors can serve as both causes and consequences of this disorder. First, there is strong evidence showing that ADHD tends to run in families and that multiple genes may be involved in the etiology of symptoms (Nigg, 2006). In fact, investigations of twins reared apart and adoption studies have consistently yielded high heritability estimates (> 80%) for parent-rated ADHD symptoms, with these estimates being as high as those obtained for height and IQ (Barkley, 2006). Significant associations between ADHD and several candidate genes (e.g., *DAT1, DRD4, 5HTT*) have been found supporting the hypothesis that multiple genes are etiologically involved (Gizer, Ficks, & Waldman, 2009).

Although biological factors play the largest role in accounting for ADHD symptoms, familial interactions and related environmental events also may account for some variance, particularly in relation to the development of comorbid antisocial behavior. For example, Patterson's theory of the development of antisocial behavior (Patterson, Reid, & Dishion, 1992) is that it begins in the home during the toddler/preschool years. Specifically, children learn that aversive behavior (e.g., crying, defiance) turns off the aversive behavior of parents (e.g., commands). Over repeated trials, children learn to use aversive behaviors as a method to control unpleasant and chaotic situations (Dishion, Patterson, & Kavanagh, 1992). As children develop, these coercive exchanges intensify in frequency and severity, persist over time, generalize across settings, and result in rejection by parents and peers (Reid & Eddy, 1997). The major variable underlying this coercive process is parents' skill and effectiveness in setting limits and monitoring children's behavior (Dishion et al., 1992). Symptoms of ADHD are significantly associated with disrupted family management practices and can increase the probability of coercive parent–child exchanges that lead to chronic antisocial behavior (Dishion & Patterson, 1997).

In turn, the symptomatic behaviors of ADHD have the potential to significantly disrupt typical family interactions. Many studies have shown that the presence of a child with ADHD is associated with higher than average levels of parental—particularly maternal—stress (e.g., DuPaul, McGoey, Eckert, & VanBrakle, 2001), as well as lower levels of both social support and quality of life (Lange et al., 2005). The stress associated with parenting a child with ADHD not only affects parental ability to manage behavior but also impacts marital and sibling relationships (Barkley, 2006). Furthermore, parents of children with ADHD may be at higher than average risk for depression or anxiety disorders (Chronis et al., 2003). Thus, family life for those with ADHD often is chaotic, disorganized, and fraught with conflict. To the extent that marital discord leads to divorce, there is evidence that children with ADHD whose parents are divorced have more severe symptoms, exhibit more externalizing/internalizing behaviors, and have poorer social functioning (Heckel, Clarke, Barry, Selikowitz, & McCarthy, 2009).

Given the critical and reciprocal impact of family life and ADHD, the purpose of this chapter is to discuss the family's role in identification and treatment of this disorder. First, we provide a rationale for the family to be centrally involved in the diagnosis and management of ADHD across home and school settings. Second, a family-centered approach to medical treatment is described with an emphasis on clear, consistent communication between parents and health care providers. Next, the family's role in advocating for and supporting appropriate educational services for children with ADHD is delineated. Once again, the emphasis is on parent–school collaboration and communication. Finally, we consider the role that culture and ethnicity play in how families view ADHD and its treatment.

Rationale for the Family's Role in Diagnosis and Treatment

The family has a central role in both the diagnosis and treatment of ADHD. In terms of diagnostic assessment, there is no objective test or series of medical procedures that definitively identifies children and adolescents with ADHD. Thus, the diagnosis is based on parent and teacher reports of current and past symptoms along with observations of child behavior (see Chapters 3 and 4 on screening and diagnosis, respectively). Parents are in an ideal position to contribute to the diagnostic evaluation for several reasons. First, they have the opportunity to observe symptomatic behaviors in home and community settings. Second, parents are able to report on behavior from an historical perspective, which is critical given that *Diagnostic and Statistical Manual of Mental Disorders, Fourth Edition, Text Revision* (*DSM-IV-TR*; American Psychiatric Association [APA], 2000) requires symptoms to be evident from an early age (i.e., prior to the age of 7). Third, parents can provide information regarding the medical, developmental, family, and educational histories of their children. This background information is important for placing ADHD symptoms in a developmental context and establishing whether symptoms are related to prior medical conditions and/or familial influences. Finally, parents can report on prior attempts at intervention to identify what strategies have worked and those that have not been successful. Important information can be gleaned regarding possible treatment directions and the family's overall motivation to implement home-based interventions.

Of course, family input to the diagnostic evaluation has several limitations. Chief among these limitations is that parents do not observe children's behavior in school and may not provide reliable information about educational and social functioning in the school environment. Furthermore, depending on their prior experience with children, parents may not have adequate knowledge about child development and appropriate behavioral expectations for different age levels. This lack of experience and knowledge is particularly possible when the identified patient is an only child or the oldest child in a family. Thus, parent information must be supplemented with teacher report and other data in order to conduct a reliable and valid diagnostic assessment.

Parents and the family as a whole are integral members of the ADHD treatment team. Although there are many compelling reasons why parents need to be involved in intervention, several of the most important reasons are highlighted here. As discussed in Chapter 6, no treatment for ADHD is sufficient in isolation nor is there any cure. The treatments that are most effective are those that are applied at the "point of performance" (i.e., the time and setting where the behavior of interest occurs; Goldstein & Goldstein, 1998). Thus, in addition to medication, psychosocial treatments that are implemented at the "point of performance" are optimal, thereby necessitating parents and teachers take on the "therapist" role. In addition, the way that parents interact with their children can shape the nature of their peer relations at school. For example, Hurt, Hoza, and Pelham (2007) found that higher levels of paternal warmth were associated with greater peer acceptance and better social functioning for boys with ADHD.

ADHD symptoms also impact family functioning to a significant degree, primarily through the coercive process described previously. The major variable underlying this coercive interchange between parent and child is parents' skill and effectiveness in setting limits and monitoring children's behavior (Dishion et al., 1992). Symptoms of ADHD are significantly associated with disrupted family management practices and can increase the probability of coercive parent–child exchanges (Dishion & Patterson, 1997). The key to changing this coercive interaction pattern is to alter parental disciplinary practices, including reducing the frequency of coercive exchanges (while concomitantly increasing positive exchanges) between parents and children. Furthermore, parents must be encouraged to consistently monitor their children to prevent antisocial behavior (e.g., physical aggression) and to prevent accidental injuries. Thus, parent education in behavior management is a critical component of the treatment plan for children with ADHD.

The manner in which families manage and cope with their children's ADHD plays a major role in determining treatment outcome. Qualitative research has identified four potential family management styles associated with ADHD (Kendall & Shelton, 2003): chaotic, ADHD controlled, surviving, and reinvested (see Table 7.1). This model of family management style is hierarchical with chaotic families (i.e., characterized by high levels of stress and disorder) being the lowest functioning and reinvested families (i.e., characterized by use of adaptive coping strategies) being the highest functioning. Although research explicating this family management model is in its early stages, Conlon and colleagues (2008) have demonstrated that family management style can be reliably identified in families of children with ADHD and that treatment helps the majority of families move to a higher functioning management style.

Family–school collaboration is a critical and universal component to achieving educational success (Christenson, Rounds, & Franklin, 1992). The need for this collaboration is even greater for children with ADHD whose behavioral symptoms significantly impair academic and social functioning. Students with ADHD often exhibit difficulties completing homework and long-term school assignments (DuPaul & Stoner, 2003). Thus, parents are in an ideal position not only to implement interventions to address homework difficulties but also to work directly with teachers and other school personnel to support the

Table 7.1.   Management styles in families of children with attention-deficit/hyperactivity disorder (ADHD)

Family management style	Definition
Chaotic	This style is characterized by disorder and stress, as the family receives minimal external support. General lack of responsiveness to the child's needs alternates with very rigid management strategies.
ADHD controlled	This style is characterized by centralization of the child's ADHD, wherein inappropriate behaviors are ignored, reinforced, or excused. The family is exhausted, powerless, and hopeless as a consequence of the child's disorder.
Surviving	Parents focus on other aspects of family life beyond the child's ADHD while profiting from social support and mental health intervention. Parents use a variety of effective management strategies and are able to separate their experiences from their child's difficulties.
Reinvested	Parents express positive energy in addressing the child's ADHD by using adaptive coping strategies to maintain control.

Sources: Conlon et al. (2008); Kendall & Shelton (2003).

enhancement of children's academic and social performance. Given that ADHD symptoms are chronic and likely to be exhibited across school years, parents can serve as integral members of the school intervention team while advocating for their children's needs across grade levels and classroom teachers.

Given the important and complex contributions of family functioning to understanding, identifying, and treating ADHD, it is clear that multiple parent and family factors (e.g., parent–child relationship quality, marital interactions, and general family relationships) should be considered when planning and measuring outcomes of treatment for ADHD (Cunningham, 2007). These factors are critical to the development of a family-centered approach to medical management as well as to fostering home–school collaboration. Positive interactions and consistent communication among these three systems (home, school, and health care) are the keys to successful identification and treatment of ADHD.

Family-Centered Approach to Medical Management

The medical management of ADHD includes at least four objectives: 1) conducting a reliable and valid assessment of ADHD and related conditions; 2) optimizing treatment with psychotropic medication, if necessary; 3) monitoring the child for possible comorbid disorders (e.g., oppositional defiant disorder and learning disabilities); and 4) safety proofing the home to reduce risk for accidental injuries and poisonings. Consistent communication and involvement of parents is critical to achieving these goals.

Parents play a very important role in the comprehensive assessment of ADHD (see Chapter 4 for details regarding assessment and diagnosis). Specifically, parents provide critical information regarding the developmental, medical, and family histories for the identified child. Furthermore, parents have the opportunity to observe possible symptoms of ADHD and related disorders across the life span of the child. This perspective on current and past symptoms allows clinicians to determine whether a child's behaviors meet *DSM-IV-TR* criteria for age of onset and consistency of difficulties for over 6 months. Thus, it is imperative that parents cooperate with diagnostic interviews and completion of behavior rating scales in order for reliable and valid diagnostic decisions to occur.

If a child is determined to have ADHD, then physicians typically discuss the possibility of medication treatment with the family. Parents must be provided with accurate, up-to-date information regarding medication choices as well as the advantages and limitations of pharmacotherapy. They should be encouraged to voice their honest opinions about the need for medication and to ask any questions that may help them with their decision. Once a decision to try medication is made, then parents should provide anecdotal information and behavior ratings to document the degree to which a specific dosage of medication reduces ADHD symptoms and/or enhances home functioning. Parents may be in the best position to observe for any adverse side effects of the medication, particularly reduction of appetite and insomnia; thus, ratings of side effects both prior to and following medication should be obtained. Finally, in some cases, parents may serve as a liaison between the physician and school by facilitating the collection of teacher ratings as medication is evaluated.

Regardless of whether psychotropic medication is part of the treatment plan, clinicians should ensure that parents receive some form of training in behavior management (see Chapter 6). As discussed previously, family interaction patterns (e.g., coercive interchanges) and parental disciplinary practices play a significant role in determining whether antisocial and aggressive behavior develops. Parents must be fully informed of the risks for antisocial behavior and provided with a clear rationale for participation in parent education. The risks for antisocial behavior are particularly prominent in families where one or both parents may have ADHD themselves and as a function of this disorder have difficulties with consistent, clear household routines and rules. Health care professionals must either provide parent training in behavior management as part of their practice or refer families to those in the community (e.g., clinical child psychologists) who conduct behavior therapy with this population. Parents need to be prepared for the reality that implementing behavioral interventions will not be easy, but that these techniques will be critical to the long-term development of their children, particularly in terms of reducing risk for more problematic behavior (Pelham & Fabiano, 2008).

As noted in previous chapters, children with ADHD are at higher than average risk for developing comorbid disorders, chiefly disruptive behavior disorders (i.e., oppositional-defiant disorder and conduct disorder), learning disabilities, and mood and anxiety disorders. Thus, clinicians must monitor children for evidence of comorbidities on a regular basis. Parents should be encouraged to report any new behavior or learning difficulties as soon as they arise. If possible comorbidities are evident, parents will be asked to provide diagnostic information in the context of interviews and/or behavior rating scales.

Because of the frequent difficulties with impulsivity and inattention associated with ADHD, children with this disorder are more prone to accidental injuries and poisonings than typically developing children (e.g., Lahey et al., 2004). In similar fashion, adolescents and young adults with this disorder may be at higher than average risk for automobile accidents (for review, see Barkley, 2006). Thus, parents must be alerted to the physical risks posed by this disorder and encouraged to safety proof the home environment. For example, all potentially poisonous liquids (e.g., detergent, insecticide) should be stored in places that children cannot reach and electrical outlets should be covered to prevent accidental electrocution. The Injury Prevention Program (American Academy of Pediatrics, 1999) is a particularly helpful resource for families with regards to safety strategies. Parents of adolescents should be educated about the driving risks associated with ADHD (Barkley, 2004). We recommend that parents talk with their teens about delaying obtaining their driver's license. A longer period of driver training and practice may be warranted prior to allowing adolescents with ADHD to drive independently.

Family–School Collaboration

To optimize educational outcomes, parents should be integrally involved in children's schooling in a variety of ways. The most important roles for parents include serving as an advocate for their children's rights, participating in evaluations to determine the need for educational accommodations and/or special education services, collaborating and communicating with school personnel as part of school-based and home–school interventions, and supporting completion of homework and long-term academic assignments. Clinicians must support parents in adopting these various roles, particularly for those families who have had negative experiences with schools and/or who are not cognizant of the need for parental involvement in their children's schooling.

A primary role for parents in supporting their children's education is to advocate for rights and accommodations under Section 504 of the Rehabilitation Act of 1973 (PL 93-112) and the Individuals with Disabilities Education Act (IDEA) of 2004 (PL 108-446). Section 504 is a federal civil rights regulation mandating that public schools (and all organizations that receive federal monies) provide appropriate education to children regardless of their disability status. The IDEA is federal legislation mandating the provision of special education for those students who qualify for services. In order to be effective advocates, parents must know their rights and their children's rights under federal and state guidelines. Clinicians should assist parents in obtaining resources that can support effective advocacy (see Jensen, 2004). In some instances, parents may need an expert advocate to accompany the family to school meetings, particularly when home–school relations have been contentious.

As part of the IDEA identification process, parents typically are asked to provide information about children's developmental histories, home behavior, and social relationships. Thus, the family's role in a school-based evaluation is to participate honestly and actively in completing interviews and/or behavior rating scales. When evaluations are conducted properly, parents are integral members of the assessment team and should be accorded the respect and deference related to their status as "experts" on the child's history and home behavior. Once evaluation data are collected, parents should also actively participate in the 1) decision as to whether special education services are necessary and 2) the formulation of a school-based treatment plan, regardless of whether special education is provided. Once again, parents may have to serve as advocates for their children if disagreements arise regarding whether services are required and the nature (i.e., type, frequency, intensity) of proffered services.

The primary focus of school-based interventions is to reduce ADHD-related behaviors and enhance both academic and social functioning (for details of school interventions, see Chapter 8). It is usually helpful for school-based strategies to be supplemented with structured home–school communication that occurs on a regular basis. The most common example of home–school communication is the use of a daily report card where students receive reinforcement at home for meeting performance goals at school (see Chapter 8). For a structured home–school communication program to work, parents must be involved from the inception. Specifically, parents should work with the child's teacher(s) to identify realistic classroom performance goals (e.g., follow class rules, complete work, get along with others) as well as home-based reinforcers that would motivate the child. Once the daily report card system is implemented, the parents and teachers would meet periodically to evaluate progress and make changes to the report card, as necessary. This reinforcement-based system could be challenging for parents to implement on a consistent basis. Thus, clinicians should increase the probability that parents will be invested in implementation by including parental input in the design and ongoing modification of the report card. It is particularly important for parents to realize that home-based reinforcement must be provided to children based on school performance, even when children may not be exhibiting appropriate behavior at home. Stated differently, parents need to fulfill their side of the "contract" on a regular basis in order for a daily report card system to be effective.

Given their problems with sustained attention and poor impulse control, it is not surprising that children and adolescents with ADHD frequently have difficulties completing homework or long-term academic assignments (Power, Karustis, & Habboushe, 2001). Homework difficulties can be subcategorized into two broad domains including inattention/avoidance of homework and poor productivity/nonadherence with homework rules (Power, Werba, Watkins, Angelucci, & Eiraldi, 2006). Students with ADHD typically exhibit problems with both homework dimensions; thus, both need to be targeted for intervention. Several homework intervention programs have been developed for children with ADHD, and all include parents as integral partners in the treatment (e.g., Meyer & Kelley, 2007; Power et al., 2001). These intervention programs require parents to provide children with a quiet and consistent place to complete homework, review the assignment with children before beginning, monitor completion, and, in some cases, ensure that homework is packed properly for school submission. These activities obviously require a good deal of parental time, at least initially; however, parents should be aware that they are already spending an inordinate amount of time addressing their children's homework difficulties (e.g., by repetitively reminding or punishing for incompletion) and that following a structured program often leads to significant increases in homework completion that may translate into better school performance (e.g., Meyer & Kelley, 2007).

Cultural Influences on Family Involvement

Most research on ADHD has been conducted with Caucasian, middle-class children as participants, as is the case for research with many disability populations. Recent efforts to include more diverse participants have highlighted the important role of ethnicity, race, culture, and socioeconomic status in accounting for differences in perceptions of ADHD, identification rates, service utilization, and response to treatment. As a result, studies over the last decade have included more African American families; however, many other ethnic groups and cultural factors remain to be studied. Although more empirical studies examining cultural influences are necessary, it is clear that clinicians must conduct assessments and devise treatment plans that are sensitive to the beliefs, needs, and contexts of families from diverse backgrounds.

Ethnic groups may differ with respect to how they perceive ADHD and whether it is viewed as a mental health disorder with a biological basis versus "bad" behavior that is completely under children's control. For example, the assumption that ADHD is a medical disorder with neurobiological underpinnings has been found to be less salient for African American families relative to European American families (Carpenter-Song, 2009). Discrepancies in views toward ADHD across ethnic groups may be accounted for, in part, by differences in knowledge as African American parents appear to be less cognizant about ADHD than European American parents (McLeod, Fettes, Jensen, Pescosolido, & Martin, 2007). Thus, it is important for clinicians to provide accurate, current, and clear information about ADHD, including evidence that it is a "real" disorder requiring active intervention.

Ethnic differences regarding perceptions of ADHD symptoms appear to impact responses to behavior rating scales that are commonly used to screen for and diagnose this disorder. In fact, parent ratings of ADHD symptoms are routinely higher for African American children relative to European American children (e.g., DuPaul, Power, Anastopoulos, & Reid, 1998). Hillemeier and colleagues (2007) found that parents of African American children may perceive children's ADHD symptoms differently than parents of European American children who have the same underlying level of pathology. Specifically, when questioned about symptoms in the context of a structured psychiatric interview, parents of the two racial groups may respond differently, even when the underlying child symptomatology is similar. Thus, screening measures may yield different results across racial groups despite similar symptom presentation, indicating a need to supplement parent ratings with other measures. Parent screening data should be interpreted with caution because of the possible overidentification of ADHD in African American children. Ultimately, developers of rating scales may need to provide separate norms for African American children in order to address these racial differences, much as separate norms are presently provided for gender and age groups.

Racial differences in the perception and reporting of ADHD symptoms may also extend into other dimensions related to service utilization. For instance, parents of African American and European American children appear to have different perspectives on children's disabilities, who to consult regarding children's behavior problems, implications of problems for intervention, and how treatment is experienced (Bussing, Koro-Ljungberg, Gary, Mason, & Garvan, 2005). Given that ADHD symptoms may be viewed as simply "bad" behavior rather than a diagnosable mental disorder, parents from racially diverse backgrounds may seek help from family, clergy, and other community members before considering consultation with medical, educational, and mental health professionals. The degree to which a family views ADHD as a disorder requiring medical attention may play the largest role in determining treatment choice (McLeod et al., 2007). Thus, clinicians need to be sensitive to possible cultural differences in views and reporting of ADHD symptoms by addressing stereotypes and false beliefs that may contribute to inequitable access to treatment (Bussing et al., 2005).

There is ample evidence that treatment service utilization differs as a function of race, socioeconomic status, and possibly linguistic differences. Cultural group appears to interact with other factors (e.g., insurance status, geographic location) in accounting for treatment choice and intensity of services (Radigan, Lannon, Roohan, & Gesten, 2005). Not surprisingly, children without health insurance have lower levels of care across all stages of the ADHD treatment process starting with initial screening all the way through intervention follow-up (Stevens, Harman, & Kelleher, 2005). Cultural group membership also plays a role, with Hispanic and African American children less likely to be diagnosed with ADHD based on parent report and African Americans less likely to receive psychotropic medication. In fact, of those children receiving stimulant medication for ADHD, African American children tend to receive lower dosages than those provided to European American children even when gender, IQ, and other factors are controlled (Lipkin, Cozen, Thompson, & Mostofsky, 2005). Racial differences in type of and intensity of treatment may also extend into school programming as African American children with ADHD are less likely to receive special education services than European American children with the disorder (Mandell, Davis, Bevans, & Guevara, 2008).

Racial and ethnic groups differ in ADHD service utilization due to a variety of factors. As mentioned previously, important discrepancies in knowledge of the disorder, socioeconomic status, and access to health insurance surely play a role, particularly with respect to receipt of medication. The possibility of racial discrimination cannot be discounted particularly when special education eligibility decisions are clearly inequitable. In fact, distrust of the mainstream health care and education systems by families from ethnic minority backgrounds probably leads parents to seek help from trusted community members rather than clinic-based or school-based practitioners. Thus, clinicians will not only need to provide accurate information about the disorder but must also spend some time to build trust and rapport with families who may be skeptical of services.

Although not widely studied, there may be actual differences in treatment outcome across cultural groups. For example, African American adolescents with ADHD may experience significant increases in systolic and diastolic blood pressure when treated with methylphenidate, beyond what is seen for European American adolescents (Brown & Sexson, 1989). Furthermore, although behavioral response to stimulant medication does not appear to differ across ethnic groups, ethnically diverse families may prefer multimodal treatment to medication alone, perhaps due to skepticism regarding the need for psychotropic medication to treat a behavior disorder. In the Multimodal Treatment Study of Children with ADHD (MTA), Arnold and colleagues (2003) found that ethnic minority families cooperated with and benefited significantly more from combined psychosocial and psychostimulant treatment than medication in isolation. Importantly, the relative benefit of multimodal treatment did not appear to be a function of maternal education, single-parent status, or receipt of public assistance. Based on these findings, the MTA researchers recommend combining medication and behavioral treatment for ethnic minority children, particularly if children have one or more comorbid disorders.

Because cultural variables may affect a family's perception of treatment as well as intervention outcomes, clinicians need to develop expertise in working with culturally diverse families. Two strategies that may help in this regard include scientific mindedness and dynamic sizing (Tannenbaum, Counts-Allan, Jakobsons, & Repper, 2007). Scientific mindedness involves forming and testing hypotheses about families from diverse backgrounds. For example, when conducting an assessment, a clinician may hypothesize that differences between parent and teacher ratings of ADHD symptoms could be due to cultur-ally related discrepancies in perceptions and interpretations of sympto-matic behaviors. To test this hypothesis, the clinician could discuss each rating scale item with parents and teachers to ascertain their thoughts behind each item response. Dynamic sizing involves know-ing when it is appropriate to apply knowledge of a family's culture to interpretation of the child's behavior. For instance, sometimes when conducting parent training in behavior management with African American families, clinicians need to understand cultural differences in parenting practices including the potential for more frequent use of authoritarian discipline, including physical punishment, in African American families (e.g., Pinderhughes, Dodge, Bates, Petit, & Zelli, 2000). If this assumption appears true for a given family, then sensitive, nonjudgmental discussion regarding the limits of physical punishment relative to the merits of positive reinforcement should ensue.

Possible cultural differences are especially important when con-sidering parent training as part of the treatment plan. Most parent training programs have been developed using assumptions from a European American "middle-class" viewpoint—assumptions that may be less relevant for ethnically, linguistically, and socioeconomically diverse families. As stated previously, cultures may differ with respect to preferred disciplinary practices. Another important issue is the inclusion of family members beyond the mother when conducting parent training. In some cultures, it may be particularly critical for fathers and/or extended family members to attend sessions, find the treatment acceptable, and implement suggested parenting strategies. Adjustments to parent training strategies might be necessary to fully engage fathers and other family members. For example, Fabiano and colleagues (2009) found that fathers of children with ADHD were more likely to be engaged and satisfied with behavioral parent training that included a sports skills coaching component than a more typical par-ent training approach.

It is also important to consider the impact of family situations on the identification and treatment of children with ADHD. Several studies have indicated that adopted children and adolescents are more likely to have ADHD than nonadopted youths. For example, in a large sample of adopted youths, Simmel and colleagues (2001) found that over 20% of children exhibited significant symptoms of ADHD—a prevalence rate that is approximately four times higher than in the gen-eral population. Adopted children who were exposed to preadoption abuse and neglect, experienced prenatal drug exposure, were adopted later in life, and/or who were placed in multiple foster homes before adoption were at greatest risk for ADHD and disruptive behavior disorder symptomatology. The impact of foster care placement has been documented in studies indicating that mental disorders in general are more prominent in foster children (dosReis, Zito, Safer, & Soeken, 2001) and that children in foster care are more likely to have one or more coexisting psychiatric disorders (dosReis, Owens, Puccia, & Leaf, 2004). The most prevalent disorders among youths in foster care are ADHD, depression, and developmental disorders (dosReis et al., 2001). As a function of the increased prevalence of ADHD and comorbid disorders, youths in foster care are significantly more likely to be placed on complex psychopharmacological regimens (dosReis et al., 2004) and to receive mental health services (dosReis et al., 2001) than children in the general population.

Given the relatively higher rate of ADHD and associated psychiatric disorders among adopted children and youth in foster care, clinicians need to be more vigilant for symptoms of this disorder in this population and may need to implement more intensive, multimodal treatment approaches. Specifically, screening for ADHD should be conducted early in life and on a regular basis for children in foster care or adoptive families. Furthermore, screening measures for possible comorbid conditions, especially the other disruptive behavior disorders and depression, should be included. Also, given the multiple complications that could be evident as a function of disrupted family life and comorbid psychiatric conditions, a combined treatment approach including medication and intensive behavior modification will need to be considered in many cases. There is no evidence to suggest that children in foster care or adoptive families are any less responsive to standard ADHD treatments; however, they may need more intensive, combined approaches than children with ADHD in the general population because of possible inconsistencies in parental discipline across foster placements.

Conclusions

Although neurobiological factors account for the majority of variance in ADHD symptoms, familial interactions and parent disciplinary practices play a strong role in determining the severity of symptoms, as well as affect the risk for comorbid disruptive behavior disorders. Thus, parents have many important roles in the management of ADHD as they are integrally involved in the screening, diagnosis, medical management, educational programming, and psychosocial treatment of this disorder. Health care and education professionals must respect parents as "experts" regarding the development and home behavior of their children while providing opportunities for parental input into all treatment decision making. After all, parents will be in the best position to deliver interventions at the critical "point of performance" and are therefore their children's primary therapists. Thus, clinicians need to provide families with current, accurate, data-based information about the disorder and its treatment so that parents are in the best position to help their children. Furthermore, assessment and intervention need to be sensitive to individual family backgrounds and situations, especially as these factors may affect perceptions and knowledge of the disorder. Ultimately, parents need to be treated as fully informed partners in the management of their children's ADHD throughout their development.

References

American Academy of Pediatrics. (1999). *TIPP—The injury prevention program.* Elk Grove Village, IL: Author.

American Psychiatric Association. (2000). *Diagnostic and statistical manual of mental disorders* (4th ed., Text rev.). Washington, DC: Author.

Arnold, L.E., Elliott, M., Sachs, L., Kraemer, H.C., Abikoff, H.B., Conners, C.K., et al. (2003). Effects of ethnicity on treatment attendance, stimulant response/dose, and 14-month outcome in ADHD. *Journal of Consulting and Clinical Psychology, 71,* 713–727.

Barkley, R. (2004). Driving impairments in teens and adults with attention-deficit/hyperactivity disorder. *Psychiatric Clinics of North America, 27,* 233–260.

Barkley, R.A. (Ed.). (2006). *Attention-deficit/hyperactivity disorder: A handbook for diagnosis and treatment* (3rd ed.). New York: Guilford Press.

Brown, R.T., & Sexson, S.B. (1989). Effects of methylphenidate on cardiovascular responses in attention deficit hyperactivity disordered adolescents. *Journal of Adolescent Health Care, 10,* 179–183.

Bussing, R., Koro-Ljungberg, M.E., Gary, F., Mason, D.M., & Garvan, C.W. (2005). Exploring help-seeking for ADHD symptoms: A mixed-methods approach. *Harvard Review of Psychiatry, 13,* 85–101.

Carpenter-Song, E. (2009). Caught in the psychiatric net: Meanings and experiences of ADHD, pediatric bipolar disorder and mental health treatment among a diverse group of families in the United States. *Culture, Medicine, and Society, 33,* 61–85.

Christenson, S.L., Rounds, T., & Franklin, M.J. (1992). Home-school collaboration: Effects, issues, and opportunities. In S.L. Christenson & J.C. Conoley (Eds.), *Home–school collaboration: Enhancing children's academic and social competence.* Silver Spring, MD: National Association of School Psychologists.

Chronis, A.M., Lahey, B.B., Pelham, W.E., Jr., Kipp, H.I., Baumann, B.L., & Lee, S.S. (2003). Psychopathology and substance abuse in parents of young children with attention-deficit/hyperactivity disorder. *Journal of the American Academy of Child and Adolescent Psychiatry, 42,* 1424–1432.

Conlon, K.E., Strassle, C.G., Vinh, D., & Trout, G. (2008). Family management styles and ADHD: Utility and treatment implications. *Journal of Family Nursing, 14,* 181–200.

Cunningham, C.E. (2007). A family-centered approach to planning and measuring the outcome of interventions for children with attention-deficit/hyperactivity disorder. *Journal of Pediatric Psychology, 32,* 676–694.

Dishion, T.J., & Patterson, G.R. (1997). The timing and severity of antisocial behavior: Three hypotheses within an ecological framework. In D.M. Stoff, J. Breiling, & J.D. Maser (Eds.), *Handbook of antisocial behavior* (pp. 205–217). New York: Wiley.

Dishion, T.J., Patterson, G.R., & Kavanagh, K.A. (1992). An experimental test of the coercion model: Linking theory, measurement, and intervention. In J. McCord & R.E. Tremblay (Eds.), *Preventing antisocial behavior: Interventions from birth through adolescence* (pp. 253–282). New York: Guilford Press.

dosReis, S., Owens, P.L., Puccia, K.B., & Leaf, P.J. (2004). Multimodal treatment for ADHD among youths in three Medicaid subgroups: Disabled, foster care, and low income. *Psychiatric Services, 55,* 1041–1048.

dosReis, S., Zito, J.M., Safer, D.J., & Soeken, K.L. (2001). Mental health services for youths in foster care and disabled youths. *American Journal of Public Health, 91,* 1094–1099.

DuPaul, G.J., McGoey, K.E., Eckert, T.L., & VanBrakle, J. (2001). Preschool children with attention-deficit/hyperactivity disorder: Impairments in behavioral, social, and school functioning. *Journal of the American Academy of Child and Adolescent Psychiatry, 40,* 508–515.

DuPaul, G.J., Power, T.J., Anastopoulos, A.D., & Reid, R. (1998). *ADHD Rating Scale-IV: Checklist, norms, and clinical interpretation.* New York: Guilford Press.

DuPaul, G.J., & Stoner, G. (2003). *ADHD in the schools: Assessment and intervention strategies* (2nd ed.). New York: Guilford Press.

Fabiano, G.A., Chacko, A., Pelham, W.E., Jr., Robb, J., Walker, K.S., Wymbs, F., et al. (2009). A comparison of behavioral parent training programs for fathers of children with attention-deficit/hyperactivity disorder. *Behavior Therapy, 40,* 190–204.

Gizer, I.R., Ficks, C., & Waldman, I.D. (2009). Candidate gene studies of ADHD: A meta-analytic review. *Human Genetics, 126,* 51–90.

Goldstein, S., & Goldstein, M. (1998). *Managing attention deficit hyperactivity disorder in children: A guide for practitioners* (2nd ed.). New York: Wiley.

Heckel, L., Clarke, A., Barry, R., Selikowitz, M., & McCarthy, R. (2009). The relationship between divorce and the psychological well-being of children with ADHD: Differences in age, gender, and subtype. *Emotional and Behavioural Difficulties, 14,* 49–68.

Hillemeier, M.M., Foster, E.M., Heinrichs, B., Heier, B., & Conduct Problems Prevention Research Group. (2007). Racial differences in parental reports of attention-deficit/hyperactivity disorder behaviors. *Journal of Developmental and Behavioral Pediatrics, 28,* 353–361.

Hurt, E.A., Hoza, B., & Pelham, W.E., Jr. (2007). Parenting, family loneliness, and peer functioning in boys with attention-deficit/hyperactivity disorder. *Journal of Abnormal Child Psychology, 35,* 543–555.

Individuals with Disabilities Education Act (IDEA) of 2000, PL 108-446, 20 U.S.C. §§ 1400 *et seq.*

Jensen, P.S. (2004). *Making the system work for your child with ADHD*. New York: Guilford Press.

Kendall, J., & Shelton, K. (2003). A typology of management styles in families with children with ADHD. *Journal of Family Nursing, 9*, 257–280.

Lahey, B.B., Pelham, W.E., Loney, J., Kipp, H., Ehrhardt, A., Lee, S.S., et al. (2004). Three-year predictive validity of *DSM-IV* attention deficit hyperactivity disorder in children diagnosed at 4–6 years of age. *American Journal of Psychiatry, 161*, 2014–2020.

Lange, G., Sheerin, D., Carr, A., Barton, V., Mulligan, A., Belton, M., et al. (2005). Family factors associated with attention deficit hyperactivity disorder and emotional disorders in children. *Journal of Family Therapy, 27*, 76–96.

Lipkin, P.H., Cozen, M.A., Thompson, R.E., & Mostofsky, S.H. (2005). Stimulant dosage and age, race, and insurance type in a sample of children with attention-deficit/hyperactivity disorder. *Journal of Child and Adolescent Psychopharmacology, 15*, 240–248.

Mandell, D.S., Davis, J.K., Bevans, K., & Guevara, J.P. (2008). Ethnic disparities in special education labeling among children with attention-deficit/hyperactivity disorder. *Journal of Emotional and Behavioral Disorders, 16*, 42–51.

McLeod, J.D., Fettes, D.L., Jensen, P.S., Pescosolido, B.A., & Martin, J.K. (2007). Public knowledge, beliefs, and treatment preferences concerning attention-deficit hyperactivity disorder. *Psychiatric Services, 58*, 626–631.

Meyer, K., & Kelley, M.L. (2007). Improving homework in adolescents with attention-deficit/hyperactivity disorder: Self vs. parent monitoring of homework behavior and study skills. *Child and Family Behavior Therapy, 29*, 25–42.

Nigg, J.T. (2006). *What causes ADHD?* New York: Guilford Press.

Patterson, G.R., Reid, J.B., & Dishion, T.J. (1992). *Antisocial boys*. Eugene, OR: Castalia.

Pelham, W.E., Jr., & Fabiano, G.A. (2008). Evidence-based psychosocial treatments for attention-deficit/hyperactivity disorder. *Journal of Clinical Child and Adolescent Psychology, 37*, 184–214.

Pinderhughes, E.E., Dodge, K.A., Bates, J.E., Petit, G.S., & Zelli, A. (2000). Discipline responses: Influences of parents' socioeconomic status, ethnicity, beliefs about parenting, stress, and cognitive-emotional processes. *Journal of Family Psychology, 14*, 380–400.

Power, T.J., Karustis, J.L., & Habboushe, D.F. (2001). *Homework success for children with ADHD: A family-school intervention program*. New York: Guilford Press.

Power, T.J., Werba, B.E., Watkins, M.W., Angelucci, J.G., & Eiraldi, R.B. (2006). Patterns of parent-reported homework problems among ADHD-referred and non-referred children. *School Psychology Quarterly, 21*, 13–33.

Radigan, M., Lannon, P., Roohan, P., & Gesten, F. (2005). Medication patterns for attention-deficit/hyperactivity disorder and comorbid psychiatric conditions in a low-income population. *Journal of Child and Adolescent Psychopharmacology, 15*, 44–56.

Rehabilitation Act of 1973, PL 93-112, 29 U.S.C. §§ 701 *et seq.*

Reid, J.B., & Eddy, J.M. (1997). The prevention of antisocial behavior: Some considerations in the search for effective interventions. In D.M. Stoff, J. Breiling, & J.D. Maser (Eds.), *Handbook of antisocial behavior* (pp. 343–356). New York: Wiley.

Simmel, C., Brooks, D., Barth, R.P., & Hinshaw, S.P. (2001). Externalizing symptomatology among adoptive youth: Prevalence and preadoption risk factors. *Journal of Abnormal Child Psychology, 29,* 57–69.

Stevens, J., Harman, J.S., & Kelleher, K.J. (2005). Race/ethnicity and insurance status as factors associated with ADHD treatment patterns. *Journal of Child and Adolescent Psychopharmacology, 15,* 88–96.

Tannenbaum, K.R., Counts-Allan, C., Jakobsons, L.J., & Repper, K.K. (2007). The assessment, diagnosis, and treatment of psychiatric disorders in children and families from diverse backgrounds. In J.D. Buckner, Y. Castro, J.M. Hoim-Denoma, & T.E Joiner, Jr. (Eds.), *Mental health care for people of diverse backgrounds* (pp. 81–100). Abingdon, UK: Radcliffe Publishing.

CHAPTER 8

School Procedures and Interventions

The optimal approach to the treatment of attention-deficit/hyperactivity disorder (ADHD) typically involves multiple interventions applied across settings and time. A critical component of this multimodal treatment protocol is school-based intervention addressing ADHD symptoms and the myriad of functional deficits that may accompany these symptoms (see Chapter 5). This is particularly critical because most students with ADHD are placed in general education classrooms and do not receive special education services (Reid, Maag, Vasa, & Wright, 1994). The purpose of this chapter is to describe the major concepts underlying school-based intervention, provide examples of interventions that can be used to address behavioral and academic deficits, and explain school procedures in the context of special education and civil rights regulations.

First, school-based interventions are placed in a multimodal treatment context. Second, the results of recent meta-analyses are discussed to demonstrate the magnitude of effects that may be obtained through school intervention. Next, important concepts that guide intervention development are described. Fourth, specific examples of intervention strategies are provided. Fifth, a data-based, collaborative consultation approach is described for working with teachers to develop effective interventions. Finally, eligibility for special education services and classroom accommodations are discussed in the context of federal guidelines.

School-Based Intervention in a Multimodal Treatment Context

As discussed in other chapters, the most effective treatments for ADHD include psychotropic medication, chiefly stimulants, along with behavioral interventions implemented in home and school settings. Although stimulant medication may optimally reduce ADHD symptoms, combined medication and behavioral interventions may be the best protocol for addressing the academic, behavioral, and social impairments that often accompany this disorder. For example, Multimodal Treatment Study of Children with ADHD (MTA) investigators found that the combination of carefully titrated stimulant medication and behavioral interventions applied at home and school optimized reductions in oppositional behavior and improvements in reading achievement and social functioning (Jensen, Hinshaw, Swanson, et al., 2001). Combined interventions were especially helpful for those children at most risk for long-term deficits as a function of ethnic minority status (Arnold et al., 2003) or because of comorbid psychiatric disorders (Jensen, Hinshaw, Kraemer, et al., 2001; March et al., 2000). A chief component of the MTA behavioral intervention protocol was school-based intervention comprised of biweekly teacher consultation, daily report card with home-based contingencies for school performance, more intensive contingency management procedures (e.g., token reinforcement or response cost) when necessary, and part-time paraprofessional support to implement behavioral procedures. The MTA findings clearly illustrate the importance of school-based intervention while also highlighting the fact that no single intervention (including psychotropic medication) will be sufficient in addressing symptoms *and* functional impairments associated with ADHD.

In addition to optimizing treatment outcome, multimodal intervention may be synergistic in that lower dosages of each treatment can be used when strategies are combined. For example, at the MTA 24-month outcome assessment, children assigned to the combined intervention group received 20% less medication on average than did children assigned to the medication only treatment condition (MTA Cooperative Group, 2004). Fabiano and colleagues (2007) conducted a more specific examination of the synergy between stimulant medication and classroom behavioral interventions. A within-subjects design was used to discern the single and combined effects of different intensities of behavior modification (none, low, and high) and varying dosages of methylphenidate (placebo, 0.15 mg/kg, 0.30 mg/kg, and 0.60 mg/kg) on the classroom rule following and academic productivity of 48 children (between 6 and 12 years old) with ADHD in an analogue classroom setting. Findings indicated that combining the lower

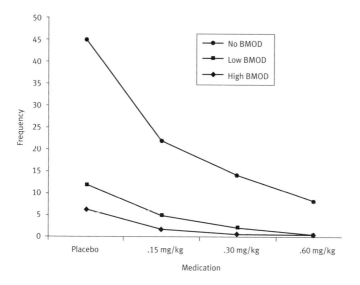

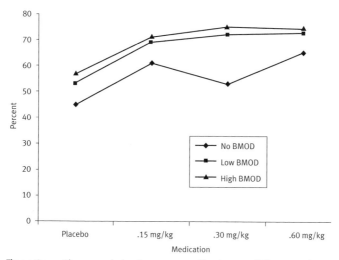

Figure 8.1. Classroom behavior measures. The top panel illustrates frequency of classroom rule violations at each level of behavior modification and medication. The bottom panel represents percent of assigned seatwork completed at each level of behavior modification and medication. (*Key:* BMOD, behavior modification.) (From Fabiano, G.A., Pelham, W.E., Jr., Gnagy, E.M., Burrows-Maclean, L., Coles, E.K., Chacko, A., et al. [2007]. The single and combined effects of multiple intensities of behavior modification and methylphenidate for children with attention deficit hyperactivity disorder in a classroom setting. *School Psychology Review, 36,* 195– 216. Copyright © 2007 by National Association of School Psychologists, Bethesda, MD. Reprinted with permission of the publisher. www.nasponline.org)

dosages of each treatment (i.e., 0.15 mg/kg of methylphenidate and low-intensity behavior modification) led to decreases in rule violations and increases in academic seatwork productivity that were equal to or better than effects of the highest "dosage" of each treatment in isolation (see Figure 8.1). Thus, a combined intervention protocol that includes school-based intervention may allow the use of lower-intensity treatment components, thereby increasing cost effectiveness and possibly enhancing consumer (e.g., teacher) satisfaction.

Magnitude of School-Based Intervention Effects

Several meta-analyses have been conducted that shed light on the magnitude of effects that can be elicited by school-based interventions for children with ADHD. A meta-analysis provides a statistical summary of effects obtained across treatment outcome studies. Typically, effect sizes (ES) are calculated to document treatment-induced change in standard deviation units. (For more details regarding meta-analysis, see Borenstein, Hedges, Higgins, & Rothstein, 2009.) DuPaul and Eckert (1997) examined 63 outcome studies conducted between 1971 and 1995 that involved school-based interventions for students with ADHD. Because effect sizes are calculated differently as a function of experimental design, this meta-analysis reported results for between-group, within-subject, and single-subject designs. Across studies, the mean effect size for school-based intervention impact on classroom behavior was in the moderate range (between-group design, mean ES = 0.45; within-subject design, mean ES = 0.64; single-subject design, mean ES = 1.16). To put these effect sizes in perspective, large effects (mean ES $\geq$ 1.0) on behavior typically are obtained for between-group studies of methylphenidate and other stimulant medications (e.g., Conners, 2002). Obtained effects for academic achievement and related outcomes were in the small range (within-subject design, mean ES = 0.31; single-subject design, mean ES = 0.82). Interestingly, contingency management and academic intervention strategies were equivalent with respect to effects on behavior, with both superior to cognitive-behavioral treatment.

Similar findings have been obtained with subsequent meta-analyses that have focused on academic outcomes (Trout, Ortiz Lienemann, Reid, & Epstein, 2007) and the effects of psychosocial treatment, including school-based intervention (Fabiano et al., 2009; Van der Oord, Prins, Oosterlaan, & Emmelkamp, 2008). Specifically, Trout and colleagues examined 41 studies conducted between 1963 and 2004 that investigated the effects of nonmedication treatment on academic performance of students with ADHD. Mean effect sizes across types of intervention (e.g., antecedent-based, peer tutoring, self-regulation) ranged from 0.25 to 2.00, with most in the modest range. It is difficult to interpret the meaning of these effect sizes because they were not reported separately for different types of experimental designs. Based on their analyses, Trout and colleagues concluded that intervention effects on academic performance are limited and certainly less than that found for behavioral outcomes. Fabiano and colleagues (2009) found moderate to large effect sizes ranging from 0.70 to 3.78 depending on type of experimental design for outcomes associated with behavioral treatment in 174 studies conducted between 1976 and 2008. Separate effects for school-based intervention were not reported; however, behavioral effects on teacher ratings were in the moderate range (i.e., mean ES = 0.33–0.78) while effects on academic achievement were smaller (i.e., mean ES = 0.11–0.33). Finally, Van der Oord and colleagues (2008) found moderate effects (mean ES = 0.43–0.75) on teacher ratings of ADHD and social behavior for 26 studies of psychosocial intervention published between 1985 and 2006. As was the case for the other meta-analyses, the mean effect size for academic outcome was in the small range (mean ES = 0.19).

The results of these meta-analyses lead to several conclusions regarding school-based interventions for ADHD:

1. Classroom interventions lead to clinically significant behavioral change that is moderate in magnitude (i.e., a change of at least 0.5 standard deviation units).

2. The magnitude of behavioral change is less than that obtained with stimulant medication; however, impact on social and academic functioning is similar to or superior to that obtained with medication.

3. Intervention impact is greater for behavioral functioning than for academic performance; in fact, treatment effects on achievement are relatively small (i.e., a change of 0.3 standard deviation units or less).

4. Effects on behavior are equivalent for contingency management and academic intervention strategies, with both approaches superior to cognitive treatment approaches.

These findings imply that treatment focusing on functional impairments—in this case, academic achievement—may elicit changes not only in impairment but also with respect to behavioral symptoms of the disorder. Stated differently, given that academic productivity and ADHD-related off-task behavior are incompatible, strategies that increase the former should reduce the latter.

Principles to Guide Intervention Development

Several principles are important to consider when designing school-based interventions for children and adolescents with ADHD. First, it is important to design a treatment plan that is balanced with respect to the use of proactive and reactive strategies. All too often when students exhibit challenging behaviors in school settings, teachers and other school personnel react to the behavior with some form of punishment (e.g., removal from classroom, detention, suspension). The use of punishment alone rarely is effective in changing behavior, especially when working with children who have ADHD or related behavior disorders. When a reactive approach includes positive reinforcement (e.g., praise or access to preferred activities) following appropriate behavior, greater success can be achieved. Yet, positive reinforcement is also a reactive strategy wherein adults have to wait for a behavior (in this case, an appropriate behavior) to occur before reacting by providing contingencies. Changing environmental events *before* a specific behavior occurs involves proactive intervention. In using proactive strategies, teachers anticipate situations where challenging behavior is likely to occur (e.g., when a student with ADHD is presented with written seatwork requiring sustained attention and effort) and modify events so that a challenging behavior is less likely to occur. For example, posting and reviewing classroom rules on a frequent basis may aid in reducing disruptive behavior (Paine, Radicchi, Rosellini, Deutchman, & Darch, 1983). A balanced treatment plan that includes both proactive and reactive intervention strategies is more likely to succeed than the typical approach that emphasizes consequences, primarily punishment.

A second important guiding principle is to design intervention plans that involve multiple mediators for delivering treatment. Not surprisingly, teachers implement most classroom interventions for students with ADHD; however, given that most children with this disorder are in general education classrooms and that the latter typically include 20–30 students, it is challenging for teachers to deliver interventions to individual students across an entire 6-hour school day. Thus, it is important to design interventions that can be implemented or mediated by others, including parents, peers, computer technology, and the students with ADHD themselves. Table 8.1 lists possible mediators and examples of interventions that could be implemented by each. These interventions will be described in greater detail later in the chapter; however, the critical point is that using multiple mediators will enhance the feasibility and acceptability of treatment plans.

Table 8.1. Possible mediators of school-based interventions for attention-deficit/hyperactivity disorder (ADHD)

Intervention agent	Preschool	Elementary	Secondary
Teacher mediated	Behavior management, instructional strategies	Behavior management, instructional strategies	Study skills, contracting
Parent mediated	Behavior management, communication with teachers	Goal setting, contracting, home-based reinforcement, parent tutoring	Negotiating, contracting, home-based reinforcement
Peer mediated		Peer tutoring	Peer coaching, peer mediation
Computer mediated		Instruction, drill and practice	Instruction, word processing
Self mediated		Self-monitoring	Self-monitoring, self-evaluation

From DuPaul, G.J., & Stoner, G. (2010). Interventions for attention-deficit/hyperactivity disorder. In M. Shinn, H. Walker, & G. Stoner (Eds.), *Interventions for achievement and behavior in a three-tier model including RTI* (3rd ed.). Bethesda, MD: National Association of School Psychologists. Copyright © 2010 by the National Association of School Psychologists, Bethseda, MD. Adapted with permission of the publisher. www.nasponline.org)

A third guiding principle for designing intervention plans is to consider behavioral function, especially when using contingency management. Researchers in the area of applied behavior analysis have identified at least five possible functions that disruptive or challenging behavior can serve in classroom settings (for review, see DuPaul & Ervin, 1996). Thus, challenging behavior could allow a child to 1) avoid or escape effortful tasks (e.g., seatwork); 2) obtain peer attention; 3) obtain teacher attention; 4) gain access to a desired object (e.g., toy or game); and/or 5) obtain sensory stimulation (e.g., daydreaming about pleasant activities). Typically, behavioral function is determined through behavioral observation and interviews with students and teachers—a process that is referred to as *functional assessment* (O'Neill et al., 1997). The central premise underlying functional assessment is that once a behavioral function is determined, an intervention addressing this putative function can be implemented such that a function-based intervention will be more successful and time-efficient than implementing strategies in a trial-and-error fashion. Although empirical support for this premise is not universally positive (for review, see Ervin, Ehrhardt, & Poling, 2001), most behavioral intervention researchers advocate the use of

Table 8.2.   Examples of interventions linked to behavioral function

Possible function	General intervention approach
Avoid or escape effortful tasks	Increase stimulation value of task and/or provide brief "attention breaks" following partial task completion
Obtain peer attention	Provide peer attention following appropriate behavior (e.g., peer tutoring)
Obtain teacher attention	Provide teacher attention following appropriate behavior while ignoring inappropriate behavior
	Implement time out from positive reinforcement

function-based (or assessment-based) contingency programs. Several examples of function-based interventions are provided in Table 8.2 and will be discussed in greater detail later in this chapter.

A fourth and final guiding principle is to link the design and modification of interventions to assessment data. Typically, clinicians use assessment data to arrive at a diagnosis and initial treatment plan (see Chapter 6). It is important that periodic data collection continue in order to determine whether the initial intervention plan is successful and to delineate treatment components that require revision and modification. Stated differently, assessment does not end with diagnosis and data are critical to making treatment decisions. For example, periodic teacher ratings of ADHD symptomatic behaviors could be collected to evaluate whether a treatment is having the desired effect. The linkage of intervention design and modification to assessment data is particularly critical because it is rare for interventions that are implemented in classroom settings to be 100% successful from the start. Practitioners are more likely to make accurate treatment decisions when using objective data as opposed to sole reliance on anecdotal reports or subjective information.

Examples of School-Based Interventions

As discussed previously, we can categorize school-based interventions for students with ADHD on the basis of treatment mediator. Thus, examples of interventions are provided for each potential mediator including teachers, parents, peers, computer technology, and students with ADHD. More detailed descriptions of classroom intervention are provided in DuPaul and Stoner (2003, 2010) and Pfiffner, Barkley, and DuPaul (2006).

Teacher-Mediated Interventions

Teachers are the most common mediator for school-based interventions, and a range of strategies are available, including both antecedent-based, proactive interventions and consequence-based reactive approaches. At a very basic level, good instructional practice is a proactive strategy that can help prevent disruptive behavior from occurring. For example, teachers should do the following (Paine et al., 1983):

1. Post visual reminders of classroom rules while actively teaching, prompting, and reinforcing rule-following behavior.

2. Frequently circulate throughout the classroom to monitor and provide feedback regarding student behavior.

3. Use nonverbal cues, whenever possible, to redirect students back to task.

4. Maintain a brisk pace of instruction so that students remain engaged with the material.

5. Ensure student understanding of assigned activities before asking students to complete work.

6. Manage transitions from one activity to another in a well-organized manner.

An additional proactive, teacher-mediated strategy is to provide task choices to students. Typically, students are given written assignments that are totally determined by the classroom teacher. Unfortunately, the presentation of a teacher-determined assignment is often an antecedent or trigger for inattentive, disruptive behavior on the part of students with ADHD. An alternative would be for teachers to provide students with a limited number of choices from a menu of possible assignments (e.g., choose one from an array of three or four assignments in the same academic content area). In this way, students are able to exert limited control over the assigned activity that presumably could reduce the likelihood that they would seek to avoid or escape the task. In fact, several empirical studies have shown this choice-making intervention leads to higher rates of task engagement and lower levels of disruptive behavior compared with teacher-determined assignments (e.g., Dunlap et al., 1994).

A variety of consequence-based, reactive interventions mediated by teachers are available. The most common method that teachers (or adults in general) use to change children's behavior is to verbally reprimand students when inappropriate behavior occurs. Unfortunately, teachers typically provide reprimands in a way that is not very effective. Specifically, reprimands may be delivered in front of the entire class, in a loud voice, with a great deal of emotion, and after the inappropriate behavior has been occurring for awhile. A series of research investigations has demonstrated that verbal reprimands are most effective in changing student behavior when these are delivered privately, softly (i.e., with little emotion), and as soon as inappropriate off-task behavior begins (e.g., Abramowitz, O'Leary, & Futtersak, 1988).

Another teacher-mediated, reactive procedure is the use of a token reinforcement or token economy system. It is well established that children with ADHD are most responsive to immediate contingencies in their environment and are less sensitive to longer-term consequences (e.g., grades). Thus, token reinforcement involves providing relatively immediate contingencies (i.e., tokens such as poker chips, points, or stickers) that can be exchanged at a later point for back-up reinforcers (i.e., preferred activities or objects). There are several steps involved in developing and implementing a token reinforcement program including 1) establishing specific academic and behavioral goals that are to be accomplished within a specific period of time; 2) choosing several situations or subject periods when goals are expected to be met; 3) providing tokens relatively immediately as goals are met in each specific situation; and 4) exchanging tokens for back-up reinforcement later in the day or at the end of the week. Token reinforcement programs can be implemented for individual children or on a classwide basis where every student participates. Studies have consistently demonstrated that classroom-based token reinforcement programs enhance the on-task behavior and classwork productivity of students with ADHD and related behavior disorders (for review, see Pelham & Fabiano, 2008). Furthermore, a more abstract version of a token reinforcement program, referred to as a *behavioral contract*, can be used for adolescents with ADHD (DuPaul & Stoner, 2003).

Several research studies have demonstrated that reinforcement programs that include mild punishment strategies may lead to longer-term changes in the behavior of children with ADHD (e.g., Pfiffner & O'Leary, 1987). That is, some children with ADHD may become excited as they earn tokens thereby leading to off-task, distracted behavior. For this reason, the inclusion of a response cost component in token reinforcement programs is often recommended (Pfiffner et al., 2006). Response cost involves the temporary removal of a token reinforcer following the display of an inappropriate or disruptive behavior. Students can then earn the lost token again once they begin following the classroom rules or meeting the behavioral goal. Empirical data indicate that response cost leads to significant reductions in disruptive behavior and concomitant increases in academic productivity—in some cases, commensurate with gains achieved with stimulant medication (e.g., Rapport, Murphy, & Bailey, 1982; DuPaul, Guevremont, & Barkley, 1992).

Another teacher-mediated, reactive strategy is the use of time-out from positive reinforcement. Time-out involves briefly isolating students (e.g., removal from desk or classroom) following the display of disruptive or otherwise inappropriate behavior. Typically, the time-out period is a few minutes and students must agree to follow classroom rules in order to return to their desk. Although time-out can be an effective strategy for reducing disruptive actions, it must be used judiciously and only in the context of a positively reinforcing environment. Stated differently, for time-out to be effective, children must be receiving positive reinforcement from teachers at an appropriate rate and should desire remaining in the classroom. If disruptive behavior serves the function of avoiding or escaping task demands, then time-out would be a poor choice of intervention because it would actually serve to increase disruptive behavior over time.

Parent-Mediated Interventions

Although parents are not present in the school setting, they can still play a role in mediating treatment for students with ADHD. The most common intervention involving parents is the use of a home–school communication or daily report card system. In this system, parents provide reinforcement at home for children exhibiting desired performance at school. There are several important components of an effective home–school communication program (see Table 8.3). First, daily or weekly goals should be specified including both academic and behavioral goals. Academic goals are important because targeting the quantity and quality of academic work may lead to both

Table 8.3. Components of effective home–school communication program

Specify daily or weekly goals in a positive manner
Include both academic and behavioral goals
Use a small number of goals at a time
Provide quantitative feedback (points) about performance
Provide feedback by subject or class period (i.e., periodically throughout day)
Communicate on a regular basis, preferably daily
Make home-based privileges (preferred activities) contingent on school performance
Solicit parental cooperation and input prior to implementation
Solicit student input regarding goals and contingencies
Modify goals and procedures over time based on results as well as parent/student input

Behaviors to be rated	Class periods/subjects						
	1	2	3	4	5	6	7
Class participation							
Classwork performance							
Follows class rules							
Gets along well with others							
Quality of homework							
Teacher's initials							
Comments on back							

Figure 8.2.   Sample daily report card. (From Barkley, R.A., & Murphy, K.R. [2006]. *Attention-deficit/hyperactivity disorder: A clinical workbook* [2nd ed.]. New York: Guilford Press; reprinted by permission.)

behavioral and scholastic gains. Second, only a few goals (three to five) should be identified at a time. In fact, it is helpful if initial goals are all attainable and realistic so that children experience reinforcement and success from the beginning of the program. For instance, an initial goal would be completion of 75% of assigned written work. Once children are invested in the program, then target goals can be increased gradually over time. Thus, with success, the percentage of work completion can be increased to 80%, then 85% and so forth until the final goal of 100%.

Third, students should be provided with quantitative feedback regarding performance. Teachers can provide a score for each goal area (see example of daily report card in Figure 8.2). Next, it is particularly effective for feedback (i.e., teacher scores) to be provided periodically throughout the school day (e.g., at the end of each subject or class period) rather than at the end of the day. Periodic feedback involves more continuous reinforcement, which is critical for students with ADHD who may require more frequent, immediate reinforcement than other students. Fifth, communication should occur on a regular basis, preferably daily, rather than following particularly good or bad days. Finally, home-based contingencies (e.g., preferred activities) should be provided based on daily report card ratings. Similar to the classroom-based token reinforcement program described previously, points can be exchanged for privileges in the home setting at the end of each day and/or week.

Many psychosocial treatment studies, including the MTA study, have included a daily report card component. The results of these studies consistently demonstrate that a home–school communication program is associated with greater levels of behavioral and academic success than conditions without a daily report card being used (e.g., Fabiano et al., 2007). This type of system is particularly effective for those students who have relatively mild ADHD and/or have responded positively to a classroom-based token reinforcement program. That is, in some cases, the daily report card system could be a way to gradually wean students off of a more intensive classroom-based behavioral program.

Peer-Mediated Interventions

Classmates or schoolmates of children with ADHD can serve as mediators of intervention. Peer-mediated interventions not only are effective, but they also have the advantage of being easy to coordinate because peers are available in every classroom. There are two types of peer-mediated interventions. One type involves peers serving as behavior monitors in classroom (e.g., DuPaul, McGoey, & Yugar, 1997) and playground (Cunningham & Cunningham, 2006) settings. Peers can also serve as academic tutors in the second type of peer-mediated intervention. Research studies have examined the efficacy of both types in treating children with ADHD.

Cunningham and Cunningham (2006) developed a student-mediated conflict resolution program that involves peers acting as playground monitors. Teachers nominated older elementary school children as school leaders (i.e., students who exhibited exemplary academic and behavioral performance) to serve as playground monitors. The investigators trained playground monitors to prompt and reinforce prosocial behaviors and identify aggressive behaviors when they occurred. Cunningham and Cunningham found that peer-mediated conflict resolution was associated with schoolwide reductions in playground violence and negative interactions. Although this schoolwide intervention did not focus specifically on students with ADHD, it certainly is a relevant treatment strategy given the risk for children with this disorder to display aggressive, negative social behaviors.

Peer tutoring involves pairing students to work with each other on academic material. For example, in classwide peer tutoring (CWPT), student pairs complete academic work in the areas of reading, math, and/or spelling (Greenwood, 2010). Steps to CWPT include the following:

1. Dividing the entire class into two teams and then into pairs of students within each team

2. Providing each tutoring pair with "academic scripts" that include math problems, reading passages, or spelling words with tutors having access to the correct answers

3. Structuring the time so that students in each pair take turns tutoring each other

4. Peer tutors providing immediate feedback (in the form of points) and error correction following each tutee response

5. Teachers monitoring activities of each tutoring dyad while providing bonus points for dyads that work well together

6. Tallying the progress of each dyad and team, with the team earning the most points applauded by the other team at the end of each week

CWPT has been found to enhance academic performance of both low- and high-performing students (for review, see Greenwood, 2010). More specifically, CWPT increases task engagement and reduces off-task behavior among students with ADHD (DuPaul, Ervin, Hook, & McGoey, 1998).

Computer-Mediated Interventions

Computer technology has the potential to enhance instruction and practice of academic material given the inherent stimulation value of computer-based material, as well as the fact that material can be delivered at a student's pace along with provision of frequent, immediate feedback. These qualities are particularly well suited to the needs of students with ADHD. Although there is great potential for computer technology in delivering instruction on new material, available research studies have primarily focused on computer-assisted instruction (CAI) for drill and practice of newly acquired academic content. Specifically, CAI has been used to replace paper-and-pencil assignments in practicing math and reading skills.

As an example of CAI in the treatment of students with ADHD, Ota and DuPaul (2002) conducted a controlled case study of this intervention with three fourth- to sixth-grade students who had ADHD and comorbid learning disabilities. All three participants exhibited difficulties in acquiring basic math facts such as addition, subtraction, multiplication, and division. A commercially available software package (MathBlaster) was used because math problems were presented in the context of a visually appealing, arcade game format. All three children showed clinically significant gains in on-task behavior during CAI relative to paper-and-pencil task conditions. Furthermore, two out of three children exhibited faster growth in math skills during CAI. These findings were replicated by Mautone, DuPaul, and Jitendra (2005) with younger elementary school age children and extended to reading skills (Clarfield & Stoner, 2005).

Self-Mediated Interventions

Students with ADHD can potentially serve as mediators of their own treatment using self-management or self-regulation strategies. Given that ADHD is, in many ways, a disorder of self-regulation, it stands to reason that interventions directly addressing this deficit may be helpful for individuals with this disorder. Unfortunately, the cognitive-based approach to self-regulation training has been generally unsuccessful; however, behaviorally based self-management strategies have shown promise in a number of empirical studies (for review, see DuPaul, Arbolino, & Booster, 2009; Reid, Trout, & Schartz, 2005). In particular, self-monitoring and self-evaluation strategies have shown promising results, especially for older children and adolescents with ADHD and/or those with milder symptoms of the disorder.

Self-monitoring involves training children to recognize and record instances of a specific behavior in order to change the frequency of that behavior. For example, students can be prompted periodically (e.g., with an auditory cue) to indicate whether they are paying attention during instruction or a task by recording their behavior (i.e., on-task or off-task) on a checklist. Most commonly, self-monitoring has been used to encourage students with ADHD to record their task-related attention, work productivity, and/or work accuracy. One variant of this approach is for the teacher or another external agent to provide reinforcement for children meeting specific goals regarding the self-monitored behavior. Studies of self-monitoring alone and self-monitoring plus reinforcement have shown that these strategies are associated with large increases (i.e., approximately one standard deviation) in on-task behavior, work productivity, and classwork accuracy (Reid et al., 2005). It should be noted, however, that most investigations of these interventions have used relatively small samples.

Self-monitoring may be especially helpful as an intervention for older children and adolescents with ADHD given that (a) teachers at the secondary school level may be less amenable and available to participate in treatment and (b) adults may not readily observe certain behaviors (e.g., preparation for class). For example, in two separate studies, Gureasko-Moore, DuPaul, and White (2006, 2007) examined a self-monitoring system for enhancing the classroom preparedness and organizational skills of nine middle school students with ADHD. All of these students displayed significant problems with being prepared for class (e.g., having correct textbook, bringing a pen or pencil to class, being in seat when period begins). The school psychologist trained students to complete a checklist of class preparation behaviors that teachers had identified as being important for them to achieve. Prior to self-monitoring, approximately 50% of these behaviors were completed across several days. Implementation of self-monitoring led to 100% completion that was maintained even when the self-monitoring checklists were removed.

Self-evaluation (sometimes referred to as *self-reinforcement*) strategies are a second type of self-mediated intervention that can be used to address ADHD-related difficulties. As is the case for self-monitoring, children are taught to recognize and record behavior; however, in self-evaluation students must also determine whether their behavior met specific criteria. Stated differently, self-evaluation requires children to determine both quantity and quality of behavior. Furthermore, reinforcement is earned on the basis of 1) behavior meeting specified criteria and 2) self-evaluation ratings corresponding with teacher appraisal of behavior.

Rhode, Morgan, and Young (1983) conducted a classic investigation of self-evaluation with several children who met criteria for behavior disorders (including ADHD). Classroom teachers developed a set of criteria for behavior and academic performance for children based on their classroom norms and expectations (for example criteria, see Table 8.4).

Table 8.4. Sample self-management intervention criteria

Rating	Behavioral and academic criteria
5 = Excellent	Followed all rules for entire interval; work 100% correct
4 = Very good	Minor infraction of rules; work at least 90% correct
3 = Average	No serious rule offenses; work at least 80% correct
2 = Below average	Broke rules to some degree; work 60%–80% correct
1 = Poor	Broke rules almost entire period; work 0%–60% correct
0 = Unacceptable	Broke rules entire period; no work completed

From Rhode, G., Morgan, D.P., & Young, K.R. (1983). Generalization and maintenance of treatment gains of behaviorally handicapped students from resource rooms to regular classrooms using self-evaluation procedures. *Journal of Applied Behavior Analysis, 16,* 171–88; reprinted by permission.

Using these criteria, students and teachers independently "grade" student performance at the end of specified time intervals (e.g., end of academic period). These ratings are then compared with students earning the number of points they awarded themselves, as long as these are within one point of teacher ratings. If the ratings match exactly, then students earn an additional bonus point (i.e., earn the number of points awarded to themselves plus a bonus point). If the ratings deviate by more than one point, then no points are earned for that period. As with token reinforcement programs described earlier, points are exchanged for back-up reinforcers later in the day or week. After a few days of success with this matching system, teacher ratings were gradually faded using random matching challenges (e.g., match of teacher ratings required only 50% of the time). Once teacher ratings were removed, the next step was to move from written self-evaluations to verbal self-evaluations and then eventually the latter were faded as well. Thus, there was a gradual shift from an externally managed system to one managed entirely by the students. Rhode and colleagues showed clinically significant gains in task engagement and lower rates of disruptive behavior with this self-evaluation system. Additional studies have replicated and extended this finding by showing relatively large effects (changes of approximately one standard deviation) associated with self-evaluation interventions (Reid et al., 2005).

Interventions for Adolescents

For the most part, school-based interventions for adolescents with ADHD are developmentally appropriate variants of treatment strategies used with children. For example, rather than using concrete reinforcers (e.g., stickers, poker chips) in a token economy, a behavioral contract would be used with adolescents. Contracts stipulate behavioral and academic goals that need to be achieved in a certain period of time along with privileges (i.e., preferred activities) that can be earned on a daily or weekly basis by meeting goals. The connection between expectations and reinforcement is more abstract in a behavioral contract; however, the connection is still emphasized and consistently applied. In addition, adolescents should play a larger role in the design and implementation of school-based interventions. Self-mediated interventions are the most prominent way to get students involved in their own treatment; however, they can also play a role in the negotiation of privileges as part of a behavioral contract or daily report card system.

Unfortunately, very few studies have evaluated school-based interventions for middle and high school students with ADHD. In fact, of the 63 treatment outcome studies included in the DuPaul and Eckert (1997) meta-analysis, only two of them involved secondary school students. Since 2000, there appears to be an increased focus on this age group, most notably in examining school-based organization interventions for middle school students with ADHD. Evans and colleagues (2004, 2005) have developed the Challenging Horizons program to address organizational, academic, and social skills deficits displayed by secondary students with ADHD. The Challenging Horizons program has been delivered in both after-school and school-day formats; it includes strategies such as direct instruction in notetaking and studying, role playing and feedback to encourage appropriate social behaviors, and homework plans between school and home. Initial results indicate that the Challenging Horizons program improves organizational and study skills, enhances parent ratings of adolescent behavior, and may protect students from academic failure (Evans et al., 2009; Schultz, Evans, & Serpell, 2009).

Consultation Model for Developing Interventions

Although one person typically delivers a school-based intervention, a team of individuals including teacher(s), parent(s), and other school personnel (e.g., school psychologist, special educator) should design the treatment strategies based on relevant assessment data and empirical support for intervention choices. At a minimum, the teacher and a school psychologist or special educator consultant should collaborate to decide on, design, and evaluate initial implementation of the school-based intervention plan. The research literature has examined several models for school consultation that might be helpful for designing interventions for students with ADHD (for review, see Erchul & Sheridan, 2007). Recent studies have investigated the efficacy of two related consultation models for meeting the behavioral and academic needs of children with this disorder.

Conjoint behavioral consultation (CBC; Sheridan & Kratochwill, 2008) is a data-based, problem-solving model wherein a consultant works with parent(s) and teacher(s) to design interventions that can be applied across home and school settings. There are four stages to the CBC process: 1) needs (problem) identification, 2) needs (problem) analysis, 3) plan implementation, and 4) plan evaluation. These stages are completed through a series of structured interviews between consultant and consultees. Data are collected between consultation interviews in order to assess behavior and academic performance across baseline and treatment phases. Interventions, primarily involving changes to antecedent and/or consequent events, are chosen collaboratively based on individual needs of students. Several studies have shown behavioral interventions designed and implemented for students with ADHD and related disorders in the context of CBC result in moderate to large effects on disruptive behavior and work productivity (Sheridan, Eagle, Cowan, & Mickelson, 2001; Sheridan et al., 2010).

A similar data-based, consultative problem-solving model has been used with some success to design effective reading and math interventions for elementary school students with ADHD who are experiencing academic difficulties. This academic consultation model involves teachers working with school psychology or special education consultants through a four-stage problem-solving process: 1) problem identification, 2) problem analysis, 3) plan implementation, and 4) plan evaluation (Kratochwill & Bergan, 1990). Observational and curriculum-based measurement (Shinn, 1998) data are used to guide selection of empirically supported academic interventions (e.g., direct instruction, peer tutoring, computer-assisted instruction). Implementation of two versions of this consultation model (one more intensive in terms of data evaluation and methods to promote teacher adherence with prescribed treatment) is associated with significant growth in math and reading skills for elementary school students with ADHD across two school years (DuPaul et al., 2006; Jitendra et al., 2007). This consultation model also led to relatively high rates of teacher adherence with empirically supported academic interventions.

Eligibility for Special Education and/or Section 504 Services

Most children and adolescents with ADHD are placed in general education classrooms (Reid et al., 1994). Nevertheless, students with this disorder receive a variety of school-based support services, including special education in some circumstances. Furthermore, students with ADHD make up a significant percentage of the special education population, including 65.8% of those identified with other health impairment, 57.9% of students with emotional disturbance, and 20.2% of students with a learning disability (Schnoes, Reid, Wagner, & Marder, 2006). Those students with ADHD who do not qualify for special education services may receive accommodations in the general education classroom under Section 504 guidelines (DuPaul & Stoner, 2003). Thus, it is important to consider how students with ADHD may be identified for school-based services.

There are at least three ways that children and adolescents with ADHD may be identified for school-based special education services or classroom accommodations. First, children and adolescents with ADHD may qualify for special education on the basis of having another educational disability (e.g., emotional disturbance). Given that ADHD is frequently comorbid with other conditions, it is not surprising that students with ADHD represent a significant percentage of children in a variety of educational disability categories (Schnoes et al., 2006). In this case, their ADHD symptoms are not the primary reason for their receipt of special education; however, ADHD symptoms may ameliorate as a function of specialized instruction, behavioral, or mental health services.

A second way that students with ADHD may receive special education services is when symptoms of this disorder lead to identification of *other health impairment* (OHI). To qualify for services under the OHI designation, ADHD symptoms must 1) represent a chronic or acute health problem that results in limited alertness, 2) adversely affect educational performance, and 3) be severe enough to make special education and/or related services necessary. Given that an ADHD diagnosis is based, in part, on the chronic display of symptoms over at least 6 months and the association of symptoms with academic impairment, then the first two OHI qualification criteria appear to be met in most cases. Thus, once an ADHD diagnosis is rendered, then the necessity of special education must be determined. Certainly, the severity of ADHD symptoms and associated academic impairment should be considered given that those students with more severe symptoms and/or greater academic impairment may need more individualized instruction and intervention. However, current federal regulations also encourage the use of a response-to-intervention (RTI) model in determining need for special education (for review of RTI, see Jimerson, Burns, & Van DerHeyden, 2007). Basically, using an RTI approach requires evaluation of student response to empirically supported intervention(s) in the general education classroom. If such an intervention is effective, then special education is not necessary. Alternatively, if intervention does not lead to clinically significant change, then this indicates a need for more intensive services through special education.

If a student with ADHD does not meet criteria for special education on the basis of having another educational disability or through identification as OHI, then school-based services may still be provided if the student meets eligibility guidelines for Section 504 accommodations (DuPaul & Stoner, 2003). It is important to note that Section 504 does not represent special education, but rather it is a civil rights code that guarantees equal access for individuals with disabilities. There are two criteria used for determining eligibility for accommodations under Section 504. First, a student must have a physical or mental impairment that substantially limits one or more major life activities (i.e., learning, speaking, walking, seeing, hearing, or caring for oneself). Second, the degree of impairment must be "substantial." That is, the impairment to learning or other life activities must be significant in some way. These criteria are certainly broader than those used for special education eligibility determination and one could argue that any student meeting *Diagnostic and Statistical Manual of Mental Disorders, Fourth Edition, Text Revision* (American Psychiatric Association, 2000) criteria for ADHD should be eligible for Section 504 accommodations. Thus, if clinicians do a careful job of diagnosis in establishing chronic symptoms and clinically significant impairment, then advocacy for Section 504 accommodations is relatively straightforward. These accommodations are generally provided in the general education classroom and include some of the proactive and reactive strategies (e.g., choice-making, daily report card) discussed previously in this chapter.

Conclusions

School-based interventions are a necessary and effective component of a multimodal treatment approach to ADHD. Although stimulant medication may be the single best method for reducing ADHD symptoms, it is clear that behavioral and academic interventions implemented in school settings are critical for addressing the myriad deficits associated with this disorder. The unique demands of the school setting (e.g., sitting still and quietly focusing for extended periods of time) also are best addressed when multiple interventions are used. Several guiding principles underlie an effective school-based program for ADHD:

1. Multiple mediators (e.g., teachers, parents, peers) must be included in a comprehensive treatment plan.

2. The treatment program should be balanced by including both proactive or preventative strategies and reactive or consequence-based approaches.

3. Intervention design should be linked directly to assessment data so that strategies can address the strengths and weaknesses of individual students.

4. Intervention should be shaped by ongoing assessment data. As success is attained, goals can be modified. Alternatively, if desired

results are not realized, then changes can be made to intervention strategies.

5. The most effective treatment strategies will be those that are delivered at the "point of performance" (Goldstein & Goldstein, 1998). For example, if a treatment goal is to improve on-task behavior during math class that occurs at 9:00 a.m. every weekday, then success is more likely when strategies are implemented at 9:00 a.m. during math class as opposed to interventions (e.g., counseling) that might occur later in the day or week in a different setting.

6. A consultative problem-solving model is effective for collaborating with teachers to design academic and behavioral strategies. Use of this model may enhance the acceptability of treatments and thereby increase fidelity with prescribed procedures.

Given that ADHD is a chronic and multifaceted disorder, no single intervention will be sufficient. Furthermore, no matter how effective in the short run, classroom interventions used only for a few weeks or months will have limited impact. Thus, a multicomponent and multisetting treatment program will need to be implemented over long periods of time, including across school years. Thus, the challenge is to design and implement school-based interventions that are complementary to strategies used in the home and other settings. In addition, this comprehensive treatment approach requires clear, consistent communication and collaboration among school personnel, families, and community-based health providers. Chapter 9 will discuss how such relationships can be achieved and how practitioners can support families, schools, and health professionals working together.

References

Abramowitz, A.J., O'Leary, S.G., & Futtersak, M.W. (1988). The relative impact of long and short reprimands on children's off-task behavior in the classroom. *Behavior Therapy, 19,* 243–247.

American Psychiatric Association. (2000). *Diagnostic and statistical manual of mental disorders* (4th ed., Text rev.). Washington, DC: Author.

Arnold, E., Elliott, M., Sachs, L., Kraemer, H.C., Abikoff, H.B., Conners, C.K., et al. (2003). Effects of ethnicity on treatment attendance, stimulant response/dose, and 14-month outcome in ADHD. *Journal of Consulting and Clinical Psychology, 71,* 713–727.

Barkley, R.A., & Murphy, K.R. (2006). *Attention-deficit/hyperactivity disorder: A clinical workbook* (2nd ed.). New York: Guilford Press.

Borenstein, M., Hedges, L.V., Higgins, J.P.T., & Rothstein, H.R. (2009). *Introduction to meta-analysis.* New York: Wiley.

Clarfield, J., & Stoner, G. (2005). The effects of computerized reading instruction on the academic performance of students identified with ADHD. *School Psychology Review, 34,* 246–254.

Conners, C.K. (2002). Forty years of methylphenidate treatment in attention-deficit/hyperactivity disorder. *Journal of Attention Disorders, 6,* 17–30.

Cunningham, C.E., & Cunningham, L.J. (2006). Student-mediated conflict resolution programs. In R.A. Barkley (Ed.), *Attention-deficit hyperactivity disorder: A handbook for diagnosis and treatment* (3rd ed., pp. 590–607). New York: Guilford Press.

Dunlap, G., del'erczel, M., Clarke, S., Wilson, D., Wright, S., White, R., et al. (1994). Choice making to promote adaptive behavior for students with emotional and behavioral challenges. *Journal of Applied Behavior Analysis, 27,* 505–518.

DuPaul, G.J., Arbolino, L.A., & Booster, G.D. (2009). Cognitive behavioral interventions for attention-deficit/hyperactivity disorder. In M.J. Mayer, R. Van Acker, J.E. Lochman, & F.M. Gresham (Eds.), *Cognitive behavioral interventions for emotional and behavioral disorders: School-based practice* (pp. 295–327). New York: Guilford Press.

DuPaul, G.J., & Eckert, T.L. (1997). The effects of school-based interventions for attention deficit hyperactivity disorder: A meta-analysis. *School Psychology Review, 26,* 5–27.

DuPaul, G.J., & Ervin, R.A. (1996). Functional assessment of behaviors related to attention deficit/hyperactivity disorder: Linking assessment to intervention design. *Behavior Therapy, 27,* 601–622.

DuPaul, G.J., Ervin, R.A., Hook, C.L., & McGoey, K.E. (1998). Peer tutoring for children with attention deficit hyperactivity disorder: Effects on classroom behavior and academic performance. *Journal of Applied Behavior Analysis, 31,* 579–592.

DuPaul, G.J., Guevremont, D.C., & Barkley, R.A. (1992). Behavioral treatment of attention-deficit hyperactivity disorder in the classroom: The use of the attention training system. *Behavior Modification, 16,* 204–225.

DuPaul, G.J., Jitendra, A.K., Volpe, R.J., Tresco, K.E., Lutz, J.G., Vile Junod, R.E., et al. (2006). Consultation-based academic interventions for children with ADHD: Effects on reading and mathematics achievement. *Journal of Abnormal Child Psychology, 34,* 633–646.

DuPaul, G.J., McGoey, K.E., & Yugar, J. (1997). Mainstreaming students with behavior disorders: The use of classroom peers as facilitators of generalization. *School Psychology Review, 26,* 634–650.

DuPaul, G.J., & Stoner, G. (2003). *ADHD in the schools: Assessment and intervention strategies* (2nd ed.). New York: Guilford Press.

DuPaul, G.J., & Stoner, G. (2010). Interventions for attention-deficit/hyperactivity disorder. In M. Shinn, H. Walker, & G. Stoner (Eds.), *Interventions for achievement and behavior in a three-tier model including RTI* (3rd ed.). Bethesda, MD: National Association of School Psychologists.

Erchul, W.P., & Sheridan, S.M. (Eds.). (2007). *Handbook of research in school consultation.* London: Routledge.

Ervin, R.A., Ehrhardt, K.E., & Poling, A. (2001). Functional assessment: Old wine in new bottles. *School Psychology Review, 30,* 173–179.

Evans, S.W., Axelrod, J., & Langberg, J.M. (2004). Efficacy of a school-based treatment program for middle school youth with ADHD: Pilot data. *Behavior Modification, 28,* 528–547.

Evans, S.W., Langberg, J., Raggi, V., Allen, J., & Buvinger, E. (2005). Development of a school-based treatment program for middle school youth with ADHD. *Journal of Attention Disorders, 9,* 343–353.

Evans, S.W., Schultz, B.K., White, L.C., Brady, C., Sibley, M.H., & Van Eck, K. (2009). A school-based organization intervention for young adolescents with attention-deficit/hyperactivity disorder. *School Mental Health, 1,* 78–88.

Fabiano, G.A., Pelham, W.E., Jr., Coles, E.K., Gnagy, E.M., Chronis-Tuscano, A., & O'Connor, B.C. (2009). A meta-analysis of behavioral treatments for attention-deficit/hyperactivity disorder. *Clinical Psychology Review, 29,* 129–140.

Fabiano, G.A., Pelham, W.E. Jr., Gnagy, E.M., Burrows-Maclean, L., Coles, E.K., Chacko, A., et al. (2007). The single and combined effects of multiple intensities of behavior modification and methylphenidate for children with attention deficit hyperactivity disorder in a classroom setting. *School Psychology Review, 36,* 195–216.

Goldstein, S., & Goldstein, M. (1998). *Managing attention deficit hyperactivity disorder in children: A guide for practitioners* (2nd ed.). New York: Wiley.

Greenwood, C.R. (2010). Classwide peer tutoring. In M.R. Shinn, H.M. Walker, & G. Stoner (Eds.), *Interventions for academic and behavior problems in a three-tier model including RTI.* Bethesda, MD: National Association of School Psychologists.

Gureasko-Moore, S., DuPaul, G.J., & White, G.P. (2006). The effects of self-management in general education classrooms on the organizational skills of adolescents with ADHD. *Behavior Modification, 30,* 159–183.

Gureasko-Moore, S., DuPaul, G.J., & White, G.P. (2007). Self-management of classroom preparedness and homework: Effects on school functioning of adolescents with attention-deficit/hyperactivity disorder. *School Psychology Review, 36,* 647–664.

Jensen, P.S., Hinshaw, S.P., Kraemer, H.C., Lenora, N., Newcorn, J.H., Abikoff, H.B., et al. (2001). ADHD comorbidity findings from the MTA study: Comparing comorbid subgroups. *Journal of the American Academy of Child & Adolescent Psychiatry, 40,* 147–158.

Jensen, P.S., Hinshaw, S.P., Swanson, J.M., Greenhill, L.L., Conners, C.K., Arnold, E.L., et al. (2001). Findings from the NIMH Multimodal Treatment Study of ADHD (MTA): Implications and applications for primary care providers. *Journal of Developmental & Behavioral Pediatrics, 22,* 60–73.

Jimerson, S.R., Burns, M.K., & VanDerHeyden, A.M. (Eds.). (2007). *Handbook of response to intervention: The science and practice of assessment and intervention.* New York: Springer.

Jitendra, A.K., DuPaul, G.J., Volpe, R.J., Tresco, K.E., Vile Junod, R.E., Lutz, J.G., et al. (2007). Consultation-based academic intervention for children with ADHD: School functioning outcomes. *School Psychology Review, 36,* 217–236.

Kratochwill, T.R., & Bergan, J.R. (1990). *Behavioral consultation in applied settings: An individual guide.* New York: Plenum.

March, J.S., Swanson, J.M., Arnold, L.E., Hoza, B., Conners, C.K., Hinshaw, S.P., et al. (2000). Anxiety as a predictor and outcome variable in the Multimodal Treatment Study of Children with ADHD (MTA). *Journal of Abnormal Child Psychology, 28,* 527–541.

Mautone, J.A., DuPaul, G.J., & Jitendra, A.K. (2005). The effects of computer-assisted instruction on the mathematics performance and classroom behavior of children with attention-deficit/hyperactivity disorder. *Journal of Attention Disorders, 8,* 301–312.

MTA Cooperative Group. (2004). National Institute of Mental Health multi-modal treatment study of ADHD Follow-up: 24-month outcomes of treatment strategies for attention-deficit/hyperactivity disorder. *Pediatrics, 113,* 754–761.

O'Neill, R.E., Horner, R.H., Albin, R.W., Sprague, J., Storey, K., & Newton, J.S. (1997). *Functional analysis and program development for problem behavior: A practical handbook.* Pacific Grove, CA: Brooks/Cole.

Ota, K.R., & DuPaul, G.J. (2002). Task engagement and mathematics performance in children with attention deficit hyperactivity disorder: Effects of supplemental computer instruction. *School Psychology Quarterly, 17,* 242–257.

Paine, S.C., Radicchi, J., Rosellini, L.C., Deutchman, L., & Darch, C.B. (1983). *Structuring your classroom for academic success.* Champaign, IL: Research Press.

Pelham, W.E., & Fabiano, G.A. (2008). Evidence-based psychosocial treatment for attention-deficit/hyperactivity disorder: An update. *Journal of Clinical Child and Adolescent Psychology, 37,* 184–214.

Pfiffner, L.J., Barkley, R.A., & DuPaul, G.J. (2006). Treatment of ADHD in school settings. In R.A. Barkley (Ed.), *Attention-deficit hyperactivity disorder: A handbook for diagnosis and treatment* (3rd ed., pp. 547–589). New York: Guilford Press.

Pfiffner, L.J., & O'Leary, S.G. (1987). The efficacy of all-positive management as a function of the prior use of negative consequences. *Journal of Applied Behavior Analysis, 20,* 265–271.

Rapport, M.D., Murphy, A., & Bailey, J.S. (1982). Ritalin vs. response cost in the control of hyperactive children: A within subject comparison. *Journal of Applied Behavior Analysis, 15,* 205–216.

Reid, R., Maag, J.W., Vasa, S.F., & Wright, G. (1994). Who are the children with ADHD: A school-based survey. *Journal of Special Education, 28,* 117–137.

Reid, R., Trout, A.L., & Schartz, M. (2005). Self-regulation interventions for children with attention deficit/hyperactivity disorder. *Exceptional Children, 71,* 361–377.

Rhode, G., Morgan, D.P., & Young, K.R. (1983). Generalization and maintenance of treatment gains of behaviorally handicapped students from resource rooms to regular classrooms using self-evaluation procedures. *Journal of Applied Behavior Analysis, 16,* 171–188.

Schnoes, C., Reid, R., Wagner, M., & Marder, C. (2006). ADHD among students receiving special education services: A national survey. *Exceptional Children, 72,* 483–496.

Schultz, B.K., Evans, S.W., & Serpell, Z.N. (2009). Preventing failure among middle school students with attention deficit hyperactivity disorder: A survival analysis. *School Psychology Review, 38,* 14–27.

Sheridan, S.M., Eagle, J.W., Cowan, R.J., & Mickelson, W. (2001). The effects of conjoint behavioral consultation: Results of a four-year investigation. *Journal of School Psychology, 39,* 361–385.

Sheridan, S.M., & Kratochwill, T.R. (2008). *Conjoint behavioral consultation: Promoting family-school connections and interventions.* New York: Springer.

Sheridan, S.M., Warnes, E.D., Woods, K.E., Blevins, C.A., Magee, K.L., & Ellis, C. (2010). An exploratory evaluation of conjoint behavioral consultation to promote collaboration among family, school, and pediatric systems: A role for pediatric school psychologists. *Journal of Educational and Psychological Consultation, 19,* 106–129.

Shinn, M.R. (Ed.). (1998). *Advanced applications of curriculum-based measurement.* New York: Guilford.

Trout, A.L., Ortiz Lienemann, T., Reid, R., & Epstein, M.H. (2007). A review of non-medication interventions to improve the academic performance of children and youth with ADHD. *Remedial and Special Education, 28,* 207–226.

Van der Oord, S., Prins, P.J.M., Oosterlaan, J., & Emmelkamp, P.M.G. (2008). Efficacy of methylphenidate, psychosocial treatments and their combination in school-aged children with ADHD: A meta-analysis. *Clinical Psychology Review, 28,* 783–800.

CHAPTER 9

Communication

In the previous chapters, we discussed the importance of the coordination among health care providers, educators, and families. Therefore, communication is central to both the diagnosis and treatment process. However, achieving successful communication is a challenge because it must entail not just family contact with a single care provider, but also coordinated communication. At a minimum, this coordinated communication should occur between the family, primary care provider, and school personnel, particularly teachers; in many cases, it must also include mental health clinicians. It is important to examine the communication systems and the barriers to communication to understand both its importance and the issues that are likely to arise in attempting to develop optimal collaboration.

Physician–Family Communication

Whether or not the primary care physicians are the individuals who are providing the direct treatment for the child's attention-deficit/hyperactivity disorder (ADHD), communication between primary care clinicians and families is critical to the caregiving process. Primary care clinicians are the individuals who are likely to provide care continuity and will have known the children and their families for most, if not all, of the children's lives. The American Academy of Pediatrics (AAP) has emphasized this important relationship in what they described as the

"Medical Home" (Brito et al., 2008; Homer et al., 2008). The concept of the Medical Home includes the principles of continuous, comprehensive family-centered care. *Continuous care* provides the opportunity for the family to develop a trusting relationship with their physician so that even if other specialists need to be involved in their care, they can rely on their primary care clinician to help them understand the nature of the problems, help them understand what treatments are required, and help ensure that they are receiving appropriate care. *Comprehensive care* refers to helping the families coordinate the care they are receiving from multiple resources covering the health, mental health, and education service sectors. *Family-centered care* means that the physicians respect the experience and knowledge that the parents bring and treat them as partners, helping them to be educated consumers who become experts in managing their children's care. They also incorporate the patients in the decision-making process as early as possible at a developmental level appropriate for the children. The choices about children's care then become a joint decision of physicians and families working together.

Providing family education involves all members of the family, including developmentally age-appropriate information for the affected children and any siblings. Topics should include the disorder, the symptoms, the assessment process, commonly coexisting disorders, treatment choices, their implementation, likely adverse side effects, beneficial outcomes, long-term implications, and potential impact on school performance and social participation. It is helpful for children and teens to understand their symptoms of ADHD and the degree of impairment ADHD has on their daily life, including strategies to address those symptoms and impairment. In addition, children with ADHD may appreciate knowing the name of any medication they will be taking, as well as its common benefits and side effects. The clinician can clarify how the patients think about themselves, asserting that having this disorder does not mean that the children are less smart than their peers. It is also important to identify areas of strength. Identifying and reinforcing the strengths of the children allows the provider to be positive, reflecting on what is good about a child who mostly hears complaints and reprimands. Older children with ADHD, in particular, can learn to be effective self-advocates and identify when they need help and how to procure it.

Education for parents includes proactive strategies that can help make their home environment more facilitative and physically safe for their children with ADHD. These changes include making adaptations and providing structure that enable the children to best use their strengths and compensate for deficits. Such strategies include providing greater consistency in their behavior toward their children with ADHD, forming daily routines and schedules, and displaying house rules in prominent places as visual reminders. Parents need to communicate with each other and other family members to promote consistency in the management of their children. In addition, it is important for the clinician to check on the parents' well-being. Parents of children with ADHD frequently are under stress and may not take into consideration their own well-being or that of other family members. Siblings may feel deprived because their sibling with ADHD attracts most of their parents' attention. Finally, as developmentally appropriate, it can be critical for parents to safety-proof their homes (e.g., cover electrical outlets, store poisons in a secure location) as children with ADHD may be at higher-than-average risk for injuries and accidental poisonings.

An element of the process of employing a chronic illness approach is for the clinician to assist parents and children/youth in developing target goals, when appropriate, in the areas of function most commonly affected by ADHD: academics, peer relationships, parent relationships, sibling relationships, and risky behaviors. To start with, families can be encouraged to identify the three most challenging areas they will initially want to work on; parents and children can then identify additional targets as indicated by their relative importance. Such an exercise will facilitate greater understanding of the impact of the disorder on each member of the family; it can lead to an improved collaboration with the development of specific and measurable outcomes. It is helpful to have the process incorporate the children's strengths and resilient factors in considering target goals and in generating a treatment plan.

Establishing measures in interpersonal domains and unstructured settings may be particularly important. Whenever possible, it is important to make progress "countable." For behaviors such as frequency of yelling or numbers of missing assignments per week, charts may be useful to record and measure improvements in relationships so that parents, teachers, children, and clinicians can all agree on how much progress has been made. In this way, successes can be built systematically and families can accurately determine progress. One possibility is to include the target goals on a single-page daily report card wherein four or five behaviors that affect function are identified and monitored on a regular basis.

Primary care physicians can review their practice and individual procedures to develop procedures that facilitate the diagnosis and treatment processes required to successfully manage children with ADHD. The steps include the following:

1. Creating an atmosphere that conveys the message that school problems and ADHD are appropriate issues to discuss with the clinician (e.g., by placing brochures and posters in the office)

2. Developing a packet of ADHD questionnaires and rating scales that have been mutually acceptable to the practice and school system, which parents and teachers can complete before a scheduled visit

3. Designating adequate time slots for ADHD-related visits

4. Determining appropriate billing and documentation for the extended visits

5. Developing a tracking and follow-up system to monitor patients, particularly if they are receiving psychotropic medication for ADHD

Optimally, the assessment for diagnosis usually takes at least an hour. However, in children well known to the clinician, assessment may require less time and the total evaluation can be divided into several smaller segments if that fits better into the routine of the practice.

Physician–Teacher Communication

The process needs to start with physicians and teachers developing an agreed-on system of communication so that children can be reliably evaluated, diagnosed, and put on an appropriate treatment plan. It is important for physicians and teachers to be familiar with each other's rules to protect confidentiality, including the Health Insurance Portability and Accountability Act (HIPAA) of 1996 (PL 104-191) for health and the Family Educational Rights and Privacy Act (FERPA) of 1974 (PL 93-380) for education. This process entails identifying a mode of communication (e.g., e-mail, fax, paper forms) and coming to agreement about appropriate behavior rating scales, management forms, transfer of other pertinent information, and follow-up forms that facilitate communication between the teachers and the physicians, as well as feasible calling times if direct discussions are needed.

These communication systems are best developed prior to children being evaluated in order to facilitate the process in a timely fashion. The physician can then provide parents with forms they need to complete and instructions on who to contact in the schools to have teacher reports and information on any school evaluations sent or brought by their parents before or at least at the time of the children's evaluation. Structuring information exchange beforehand can expedite the evaluation process, saving time and ensuring appropriate communication between the family, their physician, and the teacher(s). When students from advanced elementary or secondary schools are evaluated, information from multiple teachers should be obtained. Clinicians and schools should formulate a plan for how data from multiple teachers can be optimally obtained. For example, the team of teachers could collaboratively complete rating scales or measures could be sought from the teachers of primary academic areas (i.e., reading, math, social studies, and science).

Teachers or school personnel can initiate the process by identifying the physicians who provide a significant portion of the care for children within their school, particularly those treating children with ADHD. Because performance in school is an important function to assess in all children with ADHD, it is important for teachers to be part of the system that identifies and helps to diagnose children and assists in monitoring the effects of the treatment program. As discussed in Chapter 5, teachers provide important diagnostic information in the evaluation of children suspected of having ADHD. They are also an important source of information as to the effects of treatment on the behavior of the children with ADHD in their classrooms because teachers are usually reliable reporters of children's behaviors (Lahey et al., 1987; Newcorn et al., 1994). Thus, a reliable and valid diagnosis is only possible with teacher input.

In addition, educational modifications either through a Section 504 Rehabilitation Plan or an individualized education program (IEP) developed under the Individuals with Disabilities Education Act (IDEA) of 1990 (PL 101-476) will contribute to the overall management plans (Davila, Williams, & MacDonald, 1991). Information about response to medication in the classroom is also an important element required to achieve optimal effects of treatment, particularly because the active phase of stimulant medication coincides with the school day. Thus, teachers are in an optimal position to report medication effects on academic, behavioral, and social functioning. Teacher reports can be obtained through the use of rating scales, daily report cards, and monitoring of target goals.

Obtaining consensus on a community level among district school staff and local primary care clinicians for key elements of diagnosis, interventions, and ongoing communication is the most efficient and effective method to assure consistent, well-coordinated, and cost-effective care. A community-based system with schools relieves the individual primary care clinician from negotiating with each school regarding care and communication for each patient. The key elements for a community-based collaborative system require developing consensus on the following issues:

- A contact person at the practice to receive information from parents and teacher at the time of evaluation and during follow-up

- A contact person at the school that physicians or teachers can contact to initiate or facilitate the process

- A clear and organized process by which an evaluation can be initiated when concerns are identified either by parents or school personnel

- A packet of information completed by parents and teachers about each child referred for evaluation

- A process that facilitates the investigation for comorbidities (e.g., oppositional defiant disorder, conduct disorder, learning disability)

- A directory of community professionals who provide evidence-based mental health interventions for children and adolescents with ADHD

- An ongoing process for follow-up visits, phone calls, teacher reports, and medication refills

- A process of communication between school and clinicians, including fax and e-mail

- A plan for keeping school staff and primary care clinicians up to date on the evaluation and/or treatment process

In the case of large or multiple school systems in a community, the primary care clinician may want to begin working with one school psychologist or principal, or several practices can initiate contact collectively with a community school system. Agreement among the clinicians on the components of a good evaluation process facilitates cooperation and communication with schools toward common goals. For example, agreement on the use of behavior rating scales can facilitate completion by school personnel. Standard communication forms that monitor progress and specific interventions can be faxed between the school and the pediatric office to share information. Care must be taken with these processes to protect family confidentiality.

Collaborative systems also extend to other providers who may comanage care with the primary care clinician. These could include a

mental health provider who sees the child or adolescent for psychosocial intervention or a specialist who addresses difficult cases, such as
a developmental-behavioral pediatrician, child psychiatrist, or child
psychologist. Agreed-upon processes for routine communication can
also be used in these relationships. The AAP Task Force on Mental
Health provides a full discussion of collaborative relationships with
mental health professionals, including colocation and integrated
models, in its Chapter Action Kit (available to AAP members at
http://www.aap.com). When possible, it helps to have improved
communication systems between primary care and mental health
providers. Systems such as colocation of mental health and primary
care providers or a mental health consultation service like the
Massachusetts Child Psychiatry Access Project (http://www.mcpap.
org) enhance the communication process. Mental health services are
available in some areas through school-based mental health clinics or
as components of broader school-based clinics.

Parent–Teacher Communication

Parents need to partner with school personnel—particularly teachers—
as part of educational and intervention teams. It is important for
parents to be informed about school services that are available in
addressing their child's needs, including those provided through IDEA
and Section 504 of the Rehabilitation Act of 1973 (PL 93-112) (Davila et
al., 1991). Parents should be knowledgeable about the eligibility
requirements for programs such as IDEA and Section 504 (see Chapter
7) and the services those programs provide. Community-based
advocacy and support groups can provide information and support to
families regarding educational rights, typical accommodations, and
related services that are available in schools.

Clear communication between teachers and parents is likely to
reduce the chances of parents considering grievance procedures in
order to get the services they feel their children need. Communication
within the school between the children's general education teachers,
special education teachers, and other support personnel (e.g., school
nurse, counselor, school psychologist) is also critical. In large and busy
schools, communication between general education teachers, special
education teachers, and other support staff is difficult to maintain and
parents may get mixed messages about their children. Therefore, it is
helpful for parents to have a single person within the school who can
coordinate and clarify the information for them. This point person

could be the child's primary teacher, school counselor, school nurse, or school psychologist.

Barriers to Communication

It is not surprising that communication among families, primary care physicians, educators, and mental health clinicians frequently is less than optimal. There are a number of barriers that limit the best of efforts. In the relationship between caregivers and families, families are sometimes quite intimidated by mental health and educational personnel. Families who have had bad experiences with health or mental health personnel for one of their family members may generalize those experiences to their subsequent encounters. Thus, it is helpful for clinicians and educators to take a collaborative (rather than a defensive) stance with families and also to minimize the use of professional jargon in their communications.

The demonization of mental health services and medication in particular (Citizens Commission on Human Rights, 1987; Dockx, 1988; Laccetti, 1988; Toufexis, 1989) has facilitated the wariness that some families have about mental health services. There also tends to be a stigma associated with mental illness. People with mental illness are sometimes viewed as weak-willed people who just need to be stronger willed (Coubrough, 2008). Furthermore, sometimes parents are viewed as incompetent and the cause of their child's misbehavior. Insurance companies may deny and restrict payments for mental health services. Parents also worry about the diagnosis creating a precondition that affects their ability to get health insurance in the future. Given the limited access that many individuals have to mental health services and the stigma associated with mental illness, it is not surprising that in many cases conditions such as ADHD are not diagnosed and treated. Clinicians and educators should identify and minimize any biases that they hold in relation to families and should also play an educative role in reducing the stigma and misinformation that surrounds ADHD and related mental disorders.

Barriers to Physician Communication

There are also barriers to communication in primary care and in establishing a Medical Home. The relationship that many families have been able to establish with their primary care clinicians because of the continuity those clinicians provide is now diminishing. The current health care system frequently causes families to change clinicians because job or medical benefit package changes decrease the opportunity for families to stay with one primary care clinician.

Primary care physicians frequently only receive limited training about the diagnosis and treatment of ADHD. The assessment and monitoring processes are different than those they employ for diagnosis and treatment of physical conditions. They are likely to have received varying degrees of training during their pediatric residency in the diagnosis and management of ADHD—in most cases, relatively little training. Most primary care physicians will have acquired their skills through continuing medical education programs, so they will vary greatly as to their skills. In addition, primary care physicians are undercompensated for the time they are required to provide for appropriate care for ADHD and are under pressure to provide less time per patient. Activities such as communicating with school personnel, attending IEP meetings, or communicating with mental health clinicians are usually not compensated.

Barriers to Teacher Communication

To the extent that parents have had negative experiences during their own schooling, communication between families and teachers can be compromised. Because there is a significant hereditary component in the etiology of ADHD (Biederman, Faraone, Keenan, Knee, & Tsuang, 1990), it is not uncommon to have parents of children with this disorder who also have the condition. For many parents with ADHD, school may not have been a positive experience so they are somewhat intimidated by their children's teachers or other school support staff. Their children's experience in school can bring back painful situations they experienced when they were children, particularly if they were undiagnosed and untreated. Parents who had or currently have ADHD frequently remember derogatory terms such as "troublemaker," "underachiever," or "airhead" being used to describe their school performance. This prior experience may restrict open dialogue with the teacher and increase their level of suspicion and anger at the school system and specific personnel. Thus, teachers and other school personnel need to be sensitive to possible parent intimidation and anger while attempting to defuse this by adopting a collaborative attitude. For example, school personnel should acknowledge parents as experts regarding their children's home behavior and development while seeking their input into the school treatment plan.

Teachers frequently feel undersupported in their efforts to help their students. They frequently receive relatively little information about ADHD or how to treat it as part of their preservice preparation. As is the case for some primary care physicians, most of the training that teachers receive regarding this disorder is through occasional in-service presentations and their own personal experiences. Not surprisingly, there is a great deal of heterogeneity in the accuracy of ADHD knowledge among teachers. Given the multiple demands on the schools, there may not be adequate support staff to provide appropriate and timely assessments of the educational problems children may have. The teachers may not receive adequate support in order to make the appropriate classroom adaptations that are needed to help address the needs of their students.

Teachers and schools have been characterized as forcing children to be put on medication for ADHD against the will of the parents. This criticism has made some teachers reluctant to discuss ADHD and medication management with parents. The classroom load that the teachers must carry may make it more difficult for them to provide the individual attention needed by identified students. All of these factors can lead to a sense of having to swim upstream against a current in order to help children who have any educational challenges. Thus, it is important for schools to adopt a positive behavior support system that is schoolwide in order to address behavior difficulties of all children, not just those with ADHD (Sailor, Dunlap, Sugai, & Horner, 2009). In this way, proactive, preventive strategies are used that require fewer resources than more intensive individualized interventions (see Chapter 8). Furthermore, administrative support for teacher efforts is critical to ensure a supportive school climate and continued motivation to address the needs of all students.

Conclusions

The nature of the health care and school systems tends to interfere with good communication. The rules that help protect patient privacy (HIPAA) and pupil privacy (FERPA) add steps that physicians and teachers need to take in order to allow them to communicate with other caregivers about their children. The medical, mental health, and educational systems are all different cultures with their own language and rules. They have different acronyms and keep different schedules. These system differences lend themselves to misunderstandings and difficulties in finding common ground regarding times, modes, and content of communication. Thus, as suggested previously, primary care clinicians, schools, and other community care providers working with the ADHD population should work proactively to develop communication systems that will meet the needs of all involved. The more that communication can be structured in a comprehensive fashion *before* individual cases are addressed, the greater the likelihood of successful collaboration.

References

Biederman, J., Faraone, S.V., Keenan, K., Knee, D., & Tsuang, M.T. (1990). Family-genetic and psychosocial risk factors in DSM-III attention deficit disorder. *Journal of the American Academy of Child and Adolescent Psychiatry, 29,* 526–533.

Brito, A., Grant, R., Overholt, S., Aysola, J., Pino, I., Spalding, S.H., et al. (2008). The enhanced medical home: The pediatric standard of care for medically underserved children. *Advances in Pediatrics, 55,* 9–28.

Citizens Commission on Human Rights. (1987). *Ritalin: A warning for parents.* Los Angeles: Church of Scientology.

Coubrough, A. (2008). *Stigma attached to mental health problems.* Retrieved December 20, 2009, from http://www.nursingtimes.net/whats-new-in-nursing/stigma-attached-to-mental-health-problems/1790099.article

Davila, R.R., Williams, M.L., & MacDonald, J.T. (1991). Memorandum on clarification of policy to address the needs of children with attention deficit disorders within general and/or special education. In H.C. Parker (Ed.)., *The ADD hyperactivity handbook for schools* (pp. 261–268). Plantation, FL: Impact Publications.

Dockx, P. (1988, January 15). Are school children getting unnecessary drugs? *Sun Chronicle,* p. 15.

Family Educational Rights and Privacy Act (FERPA) of 1974, PL 93-380, 20 U.S.C. §§ 1232g *et seq.*

Health Insurance Portability and Accountability Act (HIPAA) of 1996, PL 104-191, 42 U.S.C, §§ 201 *et seq.*

Homer, C., Klatka, K., Romm, D., Kuhlthau, K., Bloom, S., Newacheck, P., et al. (2008). A review of the evidence for the medical home for children with special health care needs. *Pediatrics, 122,* e922–e937.

Individuals with Disabilities Education Act (IDEA) of 1990, PL 101-476, 20 U.S.C. §§ 1400 *et seq.*

Laccetti, S. (1988, August 13). Parents who blame son's suicide on Ritalin use will join protest. *Atlanta Journal,* pp. B1, B7.

Lahey, B., McBurnett, K., Piacentinit, J., Hartdagen, S., Walker, J., & Frick, P. (1987). Agreement of parent and teacher rating scales with comprehensive clinical assessments of attention deficit disorder with hyperactivity. *Journal of Psychological Behavioral Assessment, 9,* 429–439.

Newcorn, J.H., Halperin, J.M., Schwartz, S., Pascualvaca, D., Wolf, L., Schmeidler, J., et al. (1994). Parent and teacher ratings of attention-deficit hyperactivity disorder symptoms: Implications for case identification. *Journal of Developmental and Behavioral Pediatrics, 15,* 86–91.

Rehabilitation Act of 1973, PL 93-112, 29 U.S.C. §§ 701 *et seq.*

Sailor, W., Dunlap, G., Sugai, G., & Horner, R. (Eds.) (2009). *Handbook of positive behavior support.* New York: Springer.

Toufexis, A. (1989, January 16). Worries about overactive kids: Are too many youngsters being misdiagnosed and medicated? *Time,* p. 65.

CHAPTER 10

Future Directions

While there has been a great deal studied about the diagnosis, treatment, prevalence, and long-term outcomes of attention-deficit/hyperactivity disorder (ADHD), like any other condition many questions still remain unanswered. The research that has been completed has raised as many questions as it has answered. As a conclusion to this book, we review some of the research as a means to identify what further research is needed.

Diagnosis

The categories of inattention, hyperactivity, and impulsivity have been shown to be consistent core symptoms through multiple studies over time, and there are some children who only manifest the inattentive core symptoms (Lock, Worley, & Wolraich, 2008). It has also been found that co-occurring conditions frequently are found in individuals with ADHD. These differences contribute to the heterogeneity of the disorder. Studies have also found that some of the individuals with ADHD are associated with specific marker genes (Cook, 1999; Swanson et al., 1998). However, these individuals still only make up a minority percentage of individuals with ADHD. It has been difficult to associate any specific genes, differences in brain structure or activity, or neuropsychological tests with specific subtypes of ADHD. It is not yet possible to organize the heterogeneity of ADHD into subgroups that help predict response to treatment or long-term outcomes for individual cases.

The current diagnostic criteria are less than ideal. They are primarily based on observations by frequent observers such as parents and teachers using somewhat subjective criteria, and they do not include a developmental perspective. The current diagnostic criteria are under review for revision to the fifth edition of the *Diagnostic and Statistical Manual of Mental Disorders* (*DSM*). It is likely that the revised format of the *DSM* system will better incorporate functional abilities into the diagnosis as a possible other source to help clarify the heterogeneity. There is a need to continue the pursuit of examining brain morphology and function so that the characteristics of ADHD and its subtypes can be better understood and defined. Advances in this area may lead to the ability to develop more objective diagnostic procedures. There also needs to be further differentiation of ADHD presentations based on age and gender. It is only with more homogeneous subtypes that it will be possible to more specifically examine etiologies, understand mechanisms of action, more specifically target treatments, and gain a better understanding about the long-term outcomes.

Treatment

While selective norepinephrine reuptake inhibitors, stimulant medications, alpha 2 adrenergic agents, and behavior modification have all been demonstrated to provide short-term efficacy with more than sufficient studies (Brown et al., 2005), it is not totally clear to what extent they affect long-term outcomes (Swanson et al., 2008). All of these current treatments are symptomatic and, while effective, have some side effects that limit their utility as well as limit their long-term efficacy because of the challenges of maintaining treatments over extended periods of time. How to sustain and modify long-term treatments is still an aspect that requires further study. Rare conditions such as sudden cardiac death (Avigan, 2004) are among the long-term side effects that may occur over extended periods of treatment; these side effects still need to be studied. However, these effects are not likely to be understood until there is a better ongoing surveillance system.

Right now, all treatments for children with ADHD are nonspecific in that the choices of treatment are most frequently decided on a trial-and-error basis. Current knowledge of subtypes, brain activity, or neuropsychological activities usually does not dictate what specific therapy is employed. Ultimately, treatment is likely to be more effective when we are able to target the therapy to specific subtypes of the condition or specific brain function. A better understanding of mechanisms of action and better definitions of subtypes will be required before a more targeted approach to treatment is possible.

It will also be helpful to be able to take a more developmental perspective in treating individuals with ADHD. This perspective is taken to some extent with behavioral treatments, but most of the studies of efficacy are with younger children. Less is known about the efficacy of behavioral treatments in older children and adults. As an example, ADHD coaching (Ratey, 2008) has become popular particularly with adults who have ADHD, but there is as of yet little evidence for its efficacy. Coaching entails helping to train individuals with ADHD with the skills that will help them in the day-to-day management of their activities.

Most of the studies providing evidence for the treatment of ADHD are efficacy studies. Efficacy studies are those where the investigators try to provide the optimal treatment under controlled conditions, such as excluding most of the co-occurring conditions, limiting the age range, and having trained research staff to administer the treatment and collect the assessment measures. The studies also include a placebo condition that looks like a treatment similar to or the same as the study treatment but is not thought to be effective. The studies also include double blinding, meaning that neither the individuals participating in the study nor the researchers who administer the treatment or measure the results are aware of whether or when the individual is on the treatment or on the placebo.

There are fewer effectiveness studies. Effectiveness studies are those studies implemented in the real world under real-world conditions, in which the treatments are implemented by clinicians in the community. These conditions allow for the fact that most children with ADHD have other co-occurring conditions that are usually excluded in efficacy studies. The treatments also have to be feasible to implement when the resources are less than what is usually available for efficacy studies. As an example, in the Multimodal Treatment Study of Children with ADHD (MTA) described in Chapter 6 (Swanson et al., 2008), the children treated with stimulant medication under the research protocol (the efficacy component) showed significantly greater improvement than those receiving essentially the same medications from community physicians. After the research protocol was stopped, the differences between the groups disappeared.

The cost or the extent of effort that may be required by families and communities may make efficacious treatments less than effective in the real world. Effectiveness studies may be less rigorous than efficacy studies in being able to employ rigorous formats including blinding, randomization, or placebo controls, but they are the appropriate next step after efficacy studies to determine if efficacious treatments are feasible in actual practice.

Long-Term Outcomes

There is a good deal of evidence that ADHD continues into adulthood for a majority of the children with the condition. Most recently, the results of the follow-up studies from the MTA suggest that there are different patterns in terms of long-term response to treatment (Swanson et al., 2008). About half the children who improved initially with stimulant medication continued to be improved up to 8 years later, even when the medication was stopped. About one seventh of the children initially improved but then worsened despite treatment with medication. Better identification of children with ADHD who are at greater risk for poor long-term outcomes could also target those children who require more intensive management plans.

There has been some concern about the possibility that stimulant medications might increase the rare occurrence of sudden death from heart arrhythmia (Avigan, 2004; Vetter et al., 2008). It is not clear that these medications increase the risk, but the current evidence either way is very limited because there is no rigorous follow-up of individuals receiving long-term treatment. A better surveillance system is needed to monitor long-term effects.

A better understanding of the long-term consequences and outcomes for patients with ADHD both from the condition and from its treatments and associated co-occurring conditions is also required.

Systems-Level Issues

The coordination of care for children with ADHD is another important unstudied area. The communication between the sectors of health, mental health, and education are critical to the provision of optimal care. Attempts to enhance communication have proved to be difficult and complicated (Wolraich, Bickman, Lambert, Simmons, & Doffing, 2005) There is a need to examine the issues and try new methods that will allow and encourage the systems to communicate and better coordinate their care from the initial process to screen and identify children through the diagnostic process and the ongoing treatment process required for optimal care. It is important to determine which methods enhance, facilitate, and sustain communication and coordination across systems.

In conclusion, while much is known about ADHD with a larger information base than any other behavioral disorder in children, there are still many issues that need to be addressed to enable educators, physicians, parents, and researchers to work jointly to improve the outcomes for children diagnosed with the condition.

References

Avigan, M. (2004). *Review of AERS data from marketed safety experience during stimulant therapy: Death, sudden death, cardiovascular SAEs (including stroke).* Washington, DC: U.S. Department of Health and Human Services, Public Health Service, Food and Drug Administration, Center for Drug Evaluation and Research.

Brown, R., Amler, R.W., Freeman, W.S., Perrin, J.M., Stein, M.T., Feldman, H.M., et al. (2005). Treatment of attention-deficit/hyperactivity disorder: Overview of the evidence. *Pediatrics, 115,* e749–e756.

Cook, E.H. (1999). Genetics of attention-deficit hyperactivity disorder. *Mental Retardation and Developmental Disabilities Research Reviews, 5,* 191–198.

Lock, T., Worley K.A., & Wolraich, M.L. (2008). Attention deficit hyperactivity disorder. In M. Wolraich, D.D. Drotar, P.H. Dworkin, & E.C. Perrin (Eds.), *Developmental-behavioral pediatrics: Evidence and practice.* Philadelphia: Mosby-Elsevier.

Ratey, N. (2008). *The disorganized mind: Coaching your ADHD brain to take control.* New York: St. Martin Press.

Swanson, J., Arnold, L.E., Kraemer, H., Hechtman, L., Molina, B., Hinshaw, S., et al. (2008). Evidence, interpretation, and qualification from multiple reports of long-term outcomes in the Multimodal Treatment Study of Children with ADHD (MTA). *Journal of Attention Disorders 12,* 4–43.

Swanson, J.M., Sunohara, G.A., Kennedy, J.L., Regino, R., Fineberg, E., Wigal, T., et al. (1998). Association of the dopamine receptor D4 (*DRD4*) gene with a refined phenotype of attention deficit-hyperactivity disorder (ADHD): A family-based approach. *Molecular Psychiatry, 3,* 38–41.

Vetter, V., Elia, J., Erickson, C., Berger, S., Blum, N., Uzark, K., et al. (2008). Cardiovascular monitoring of children and adolescents with heart disease receiving stimulant drugs: A scientific statement from the American Heart Association Council on Cardiovascular Disease in the Young Congenital Cardiac Defects Committee and the Council on Cardiovascular Nursing. *Circulation, 117,* 2407–2423.

Wolraich, M., Bickman, L., Lambert, E.W., Simmons, T., & Doffing, M.A. (2005). Intervening to improve communication among parents, teachers, and primary care providers of children with ADHD or at high risk for ADHD. *Journal of Attention Disorders, 9,* 354–368.

CHAPTER 11

Resources

Attention-deficit/hyperactivity disorder (ADHD) is a chronic disorder that affects functioning across home, school, and community settings. As such, many individuals (e.g., parents, teachers, health professionals) are involved in the assessment and treatment of children and adolescents with this disorder. Thus, it is important that everyone involved have access to accurate and timely information about the disorder. Fortunately, there are many resources available on the Internet, in print, and in various other media (e.g., DVD). Nevertheless, it is challenging to stay abreast of current information given the voluminous and growing research literature focused on ADHD. This is very much a dynamic, rather than static, knowledge base. Furthermore, this veritable glut of information includes many resources, ideas, and suggestions that are not research based and may actually lead to uninformed and potentially harmful diagnostic and treatment decisions.

The purpose of this chapter is to recommend accurate, research-based resources that will assist parents, teachers, and health professionals who are working with children and adolescents with ADHD. Informational resources for children and adolescents with this disorder are also delineated. Resources across a variety of media (web-based, print, and electronic media) are identified. Given the varied quality and dynamic nature of the ADHD knowledge base in general, suggestions for assessing the veracity of available information sources are provided.

Resources for Health and Mental Health Professionals

There are many resources for health professionals that provide important background information as well as guidelines for assessment and treatment of ADHD.

Background Information on ADHD

The following resources provide background information regarding the nature, possible etiologies, associated impairments, and/or course of ADHD across the lifespan.

Barkley, R.A. (Ed.). (2006). *Attention-deficit/hyperactivity disorder: A handbook for diagnosis and treatment* (3rd ed.). New York: Guilford Press. This seminal text is considered the foremost resource on all aspects of ADHD.

Barkley, R.A., Murphy, K.R., & Fischer, M. (2008). *ADHD in adults: What the science says.* New York: Guilford Press. This book provides detailed analysis and interpretation of a large-scale longitudinal study following a sample of individuals from childhood into adulthood.

Brown, T.E. (Ed.). (2009). *ADHD comorbidities: Handbook for ADHD complications in children and adults.* Arlington, VA: American Psychiatric Publishing. This book provides an overview of the myriad of complications associated with ADHD, as well as chapters relative to specific stages of development.

Center for Children and Families at University of Buffalo (http://ccf.buffalo.edu/resources_downloads.php). This is an excellent site that includes fact sheets about ADHD for parents and educators, as well as many forms and handouts helpful for assessment and treatment.

Children and Adults with ADHD (CHADD) (http://www.chadd.org). The CHADD web site provides information regarding the nature of ADHD, as well as assessment and treatment. Many helpful handouts for professionals and parents are available for download.

CHADD National Resource Center on ADHD (http://www.help4adhd.org). The CHADD organization sponsors a National Resource Center on ADHD whose web site contains a plethora of informational resources about diagnosis and treatment.

National Institute of Mental Health (http://www.nimh.nih.gov/health/publications/attention-deficit-hyperactivity-disorder/

complete-index.shtml). The NIMH ADHD web site contains information regarding latest scientific studies on the disorder, as well as user-friendly descriptions of treatment strategies.

Nigg, J.T. (2006). *What causes ADHD?* New York: Guilford Press. This book features a thorough and research-based discussion of the variety of etiological factors that have been studied in relation to this disorder.

Weyandt, L.L. (2007). *An ADHD primer* (2nd ed.). Mahwah, NJ: Lawrence Erlbaum Associates. This is a very readable and complete resource on all aspects of ADHD.

Assessment of ADHD

The following resources provide guidelines and specific details regarding the comprehensive assessment and diagnostic evaluation of ADHD.

American Academy of Child and Adolescent Psychiatry. (2007). Practice parameters for the assessment and treatment of children and adolescents with attention-deficit/hyperactivity disorder. *Journal of the American Academy of Child and Adolescent Psychiatry, 46,* 894–921. These are guidelines for psychiatrists for both diagnosis and treatment of ADHD, with an emphasis on psychotropic medication.

Anastopoulos, A.D., & Shelton, T.L. (2001). *Assessing attention-deficit/hyperactivity disorder.* New York: Kluwer Academic/Plenum. This book is a comprehensive and empirically based guide to the assessment of ADHD and related impairments.

Barkley, R.A. (Ed.). (2006). *Attention-deficit/hyperactivity disorder: A handbook for diagnosis and treatment* (3rd ed.). New York: Guilford Press. This seminal text is considered the foremost resource on all aspects of ADHD.

Barkley, R.A., & Murphy, K.R. (2006). *Attention-deficit hyperactivity disorder: A clinical workbook* (3rd ed.). New York: Guilford Press. This workbook contains many handouts and rating forms that are helpful in the diagnostic evaluation and treatment of ADHD.

Pelham, W.E., Jr., Fabiano, G.A., & Massetti, G.M. (2005). Evidence-based assessment of attention deficit hyperactivity disorder in children and adolescents. *Journal of Clinical Child and Adolescent Psychology, 34,* 449–476. This article provides a thorough, scholarly review of various assessment measures (e.g., rating scales and direct observations) used for evaluation of ADHD and associated impairments.

Treatment of ADHD

These resources provide guidelines and recommended procedures for the treatment of ADHD. Information regarding both psychotropic and psychosocial interventions is available.

American Academy of Child and Adolescent Psychiatry. (2007). Practice parameters for the assessment and treatment of children and adolescents with attention-deficit/hyperactivity disorder. *Journal of the American Academy of Child and Adolescent Psychiatry, 46,* 894–921. This practice parameter emphasizes the use of psychotropic medication. Coverage of psychosocial treatment is minimal.

Barkley, R.A. (1997). *Defiant children: A clinician's manual for assessment and parent training* (2nd ed.). New York: Guilford Press. This very practical, step-by-step guide explains how to conduct parent training in behavior modification for children with ADHD and related disorders. It emphasizes the use of both antecedent-based and consequence-based behavioral strategies.

Barkley, R.A. (Ed.). (2006). *Attention-deficit/hyperactivity disorder: A handbook for diagnosis and treatment* (3rd ed.). New York: Guilford Press. This seminal text provides a comprehensive overview of psychotropic and psychosocial treatment of ADHD.

Pelham, W.E., Jr., & Fabiano, G.A. (2008). Evidence-based psychosocial treatments for attention-deficit/hyperactivity disorder. *Journal of Clinical Child and Adolescent Psychology, 37,* 184–214. This article is a comprehensive, scholarly review of the psychosocial (primarily behavioral) treatment literature.

Pliszka, S.R. (2009). *Treating ADHD and comorbid disorders: Psychosocial and psychopharmacological interventions.* New York: Guilford Press. This resource is particularly comprehensive in its coverage of psychotropic medication for ADHD.

Resources for Teachers and Educational Professionals

Because children and adolescents experience significant difficulties in school settings, it is critical that teachers and other educational professionals (e.g., school psychologists, counselors) possess accurate information regarding this disorder. The resources listed previously for health care professionals are certainly relevant for school professionals.

In addition, several texts and web sites provide specific information regarding school-based services for students with ADHD.

Challenging Horizons (http://www.oucirs.org). The Challenging Horizons program is a multicomponent intervention designed to increase study and organizational skills in middle school students with ADHD. It is has been implemented as part of the school curriculum and also as an after-school program.

DuPaul, G.J., & Stoner, G. (2003). *ADHD in the schools: Assessment and intervention strategies* (2nd ed.). New York: Guilford Press. This book provides background information regarding ADHD in school settings, as well as specific recommendations for school-based assessment and treatment of this disorder.

Paine, S.C., Radicchi, J., Rosellini, L.C., Deutchman, L., & Darch, C.B. (1983). *Structuring your classroom for academic success.* Champaign, IL: Research Press. Although this text does not focus specifically on ADHD, it includes very helpful information on proactive strategies (including classroom design) that can prevent disruptive behavior on a classwide basis.

Pfiffner, L.J. (1996). *All about ADHD.* Jefferson City, MO: Scholastic. Although a bit dated, this book provides a brief, clear overview of ADHD for teachers and includes cogent recommendations for classroom intervention.

Power, T.J., Karustis, J.L., & Habboushe, D.F. (2001). *Homework success for children with ADHD: A family-school intervention program.* New York: Guilford Press. This book provides a structured protocol for enhancing homework productivity of students with ADHD involving collaboration between parents and classroom teachers.

Rief, S.F. (2005). *How to reach and teach children with ADD/ADHD: Practical techniques, strategies, and interventions* (2nd ed.). San Francisco, CA: Jossey-Bass. This very practical handbook for teachers includes many helpful suggestions for teaching and behavior management strategies.

Rief, S.F. (2008). *The ADD/ADHD checklist: A practical reference for parents and teachers* (2nd ed.). San Francisco, CA: Jossey-Bass. This is an extremely practical book designed specifically for teachers and parents of children with ADHD. It includes many resources (e.g., daily report card) that can be used in classroom settings.

What Works Clearinghouse (http://ies.ed.gov/ncee/wwc/). The Institute of Education Sciences (U.S. Department of Education) provides current, research-based information on academic and behavioral strategies that can be used in K–12 settings. Although not specific to ADHD, many of these instructional and behavioral techniques will be helpful for students with this disorder.

Zentall, S.S. (2006). *ADHD and education: Foundations, characteristics, methods, and collaboration.* Upper Saddle River, NJ: Pearson. This book offers a comprehensive overview of ADHD and intervention strategies that is directly applicable to classroom settings.

Resources for Parents and Family Members

There are a plethora of books, DVDs, and web sites that provide information on ADHD for parents and other relatives of children with ADHD. Unfortunately, the quality of these resources varies considerably and, thus, it is important that parents are referred to accurate sources. The following resources provide accurate, research-based information in a user-friendly format.

American Academy of Pediatrics. (2005). *Caring for children with ADHD: A resource toolkit for clinicians.* Chicago, IL: Author. This toolkit includes an excellent comprehensive paperback book for parents.

Barkley, R.A. (1992). *ADHD: What can we do?* [Video], and Barkley, R.A. (1993). *ADHD: What do we know?* [Video]. New York: Guilford Press. Although both of these videos are now somewhat dated, they are still excellent introductions to the nature of ADHD and the treatment of this disorder for parents and other family members.

Barkley, R.A. (2000). *Taking charge of ADHD* (2nd ed.). New York: Guilford Press. This highly readable book provides accurate and evidence-based information regarding the nature of ADHD as well as what parents should expect in terms of assessment and treatment.

Barkley, R.A. (2000). *A new look at ADHD: Inhibition, time and self-control* [Video]. New York: Guilford Press. This video provides an overview of Barkley's theory of ADHD as a disorder of impaired delayed responding to the environment. Information is presented in a user-friendly way so that viewers are able to see how this theory can be applied directly to intervention strategies.

Barkley, R.A. & Benton, C.M. (1998). *Your defiant child: Eight steps to better behavior.* New York: Guilford Press. This is a concise, practical guide for parents to implement behavioral strategies to reduce child noncompliance. It is a great book for parents to use if they participate in a parent training program.

Goldstein, S. (1990). *Why won't my child pay attention?* [Video]. Salt Lake City, UT: Neurology, Learning and Behavior Center. This is another video that is also somewhat dated but a very effective presentation of essential information about ADHD and its treatment.

Goldstein, S., & Goldstein, M. (1993). *Hyperactivity: Why won't my child pay attention?* New York: Wiley. This is a very readable and accurate book about ADHD for parents. It includes very practical information for home-based management of the disorder.

Gordon, M. (1992). *My brother's a world-class pain: A sibling's guide to ADHD/hyperactivity.* DeWitt, NY: GSI Publications. This easy-to-read book for siblings of children with ADHD provides a straightforward explanation of the disorder and ways that siblings can help.

Jensen, P.S. (2004). *Making the system work for your child with ADHD.* New York: Guilford Press. This is an excellent companion to the Barkley (2000) book because it walks parents through a strategic process of working with schools, clinicians, and the health care and educational systems.

Reiff, M.I., with Tippins, S. (Eds.). (2004). *ADHD: A complete and authoritative guide.* Chicago, IL: American Academy of Pediatrics. This book is a comprehensive resource for parents.

There are three web sites that have been mentioned previously that also provide helpful information to parents and relatives of children with ADHD: the Children and Adults with ADHD (CHADD) organization (http://www.chadd.org), the CHADD National Resource Center on ADHD (http://www.help4adhd.org/), the National Institute of Mental Health (http://www.nimh.nih.gov/health/publications/attention-deficit-hyperactivity-disorder/complete-index.shtml).

Resources for Children and Adolescents with ADHD

Older children and adolescents may find many of the resources, particularly relevant web sites, listed for parents as helpful depending on their reading and interest level. Additional books designed specifically for children with ADHD include the following.

Gordon, M. (1991). *Jumpin' Johnny get back to work: A child's guide to ADHD/hyperactivity.* DeWitt, NY: GSI Publications. This book is somewhat dated but remains a helpful introduction to ADHD for younger children.

Nadeau, K.G., Dixon, E.B., & Rose, J. (1997). *Learning to slow down and pay attention: A book for kids about ADHD.* Washington, DC: Magination Press. This book contains suggestions and activities for children with ADHD to work on organization and related skills.

Zeigler Dendy, C.A., & Zeigler, A. (2003). *A bird's eye view of life with ADD and ADHD: Advice from young survivors.* Cedar Bluff, AL: Cherish the Children. This book provides adolescents with ADHD a firsthand perspective on how to manage the disorder and exposes them to success stories.

Suggestions for Assessing the Veracity of Available Resources

Although there is a plethora of information about ADHD available in print and electronic media, the quality and accuracy varies considerably across resources. Unfortunately, parents and professionals may make costly decisions on the basis of erroneous information that is not supported by scientific evidence. Thus, certain guidelines should be followed when evaluating the utility of an informational resource.

1. *Make sure that the information comes from a credible source.* In general, the most accurate information will come from reliable sources such as professional organizations (e.g., American Academy of Pediatrics, American Psychological Association) and scientific journals (e.g., *Journal of Attention Disorders, Pediatrics, School Psychology Review*). When information is touted by individuals, even those identified as "experts," one should be skeptical until determining that the information is scientifically accurate.

2. *Avoid using information that is based solely on testimonial and/or "clinical experience."* Testimonials or subjective impressions based on clinical experience, no matter how extensive, do not represent scientific data. As such, testimonial-based information, especially about treatment, should be treated with a good deal of skepticism unless data are presented to support contentions.

3. *Recognize "red flags" that indicate information may be suspect.* Common indicators that information may be unreliable include sources purporting that a particular treatment "cures" ADHD or

that the treatment is potentially curative for multiple disorders (e.g., ADHD, depression, autism; Ingersoll & Goldstein, 1993). There are no known cures for ADHD, and it is unlikely that a single treatment will be highly effective for a variety of conditions.

4. *Always ask, "Where are the data?"* Resources should always identify the science upon which information is based. For example, it is incumbent upon the developer or proponent of a specific treatment to demonstrate its therapeutic efficacy in the context of a controlled, experimental design using reliable and valid dependent measures. Furthermore, data should be available that allow direct comparison of the effects of novel therapies relative to those associated with established, effective interventions.

5. *Evaluate the quality of research upon which information is based.* Several questions can be useful in discerning the scientific quality of information (DuPaul & Stoner, 2003). These questions are particularly critical when treatment decisions weigh in the balance. Were the participants classified with ADHD using reliable and valid indices of the disorder? Were the dependent measures collected in such a fashion to reduce possible biases (e.g., behavioral observations conducted by individuals who were unaware of the clinical population being studied and the treatment being investigated)? Are threats to the internal validity (e.g., maturation) of the treatment controlled for? How generalizable are the obtained results to other children with ADHD? Was the clinical significance (e.g., normalization) of the obtained findings assessed? Did the investigators examine the generalization of treatment effects across settings (e.g., home and school) and over time (e.g., follow-up assessment)?

6. *Assist parents and families in locating accurate information about ADHD.* Parents may not always be able to separate accurate from inaccurate information about ADHD. Thus, professionals must steer families in the direction of evidence-based resources and arm them with a healthy degree of skepticism against erroneous claims they may encounter. Parents of these children may be particularly prone to adopting new therapeutic approaches given their frustrations in dealing with ADHD-related difficulties and their knowledge of the limitations of currently available treatments.

Summary

Because ADHD is a chronic disorder that cuts across family, school, and community systems, it is important that all individuals working with affected children are privy to accurate, scientifically sound information on the disorder. Fortunately, there are many resources that are very helpful, particularly in relation to assessment and treatment. Nevertheless, health care and educational professionals should assist families in procuring the most accurate information given that content quality may vary considerably across resources.

References

DuPaul, G.J., & Stoner, G. (2003). *ADHD in the schools: Assessment and intervention strategies* (2nd ed.). New York: Guilford Press.

Ingersoll, B., & Goldstein, S. (1993). *Attention deficit disorder and learning disabilities: Realities, myths, and controversial treatments.* New York: Doubleday.

Index

Page numbers followed by *f* or *t* indicate figures or tables, respectively.

PL 93-380, *see* Family Educational
   Rights and Privacy Act of 1974
PL 101-476, *see* Individuals with
   Disabilities Education Act of
   1990
PL 104-191, *see* Health Insurance
   Portability and Accountability
   Act of 1996
PL 108-446, *see* Individuals with
   Disabilities Education Act of
   2004
Playground monitors, peers as, 147
Poisonings, 123
Positive predictive power (PPP),
   30–32, 30*t*
Positive reinforcement, 79, 144, 147
Posttraumatic stress disorder (PTSD),
   58
PPP, *see* Positive predictive power
Premature birth, 15
Preschool-age children, 50
Prevalence of ADHD, 8, 13, 17–21, 26
Primary health care settings
   screening procedures in, 29–30
   treatment in, 8
   see also Physicians
Psychosocial treatment, *see* Behavior
   modification
Psychotropic medication, 76, 87–103,
   88, 127
PTSD, *see* Posttraumatic stress disor-
   der
Punishment, 72

Racial and ethnic factors, 33–35, 34*f*
   communication with parents and,
   41
   diagnosis and management and,
   126–130
Randomized controlled trials, 88
Rehabilitation Act of 1973 (PL 93-112,
   Section 504 regulations), 6, 124,
   153–155, 165
Reinvested families, 120, 121*t*
Resources, 179–188
   assessing veracity of, 186–187
   for children and adolescents with
   ADHD, 185–186
   for health and mental health professionals, 180–182

for parents and family, 184–185
for teachers and educational pro-
   fessionals, 182–184
Response costs, 144–145
Response-to-intervention (RTI)
   model, 54, 154
Reynolds Adolescent Depression
   Scale, 38
Reynolds Child Depression
   Scale, 38
Ritalin LA, 92, 96
RTI, *see* Response-to-intervention
   model

Safety issues, 123, 163
Schizophrenia, 50
School-based intervention, 107,
   135–160
   for adolescents, 151–152
   collaboration with family, 120,
   123–125
   computer-mediated, 148–149
   consultation model for developing,
   152–153
   coordination with mental health
   professionals, 1
   daily report cards, 146–147, 146*f*,
   165
   effect sizes (ES), calculation of,
   138–139
   examples of, 142–151, 142*t*
   in multimodal treatment context,
   135, 136–138, 137*f*
   parent-mediated, 141*t*, 145–147
   peer-mediated, 141*t*, 147–148
   principles to guide development,
   140–142, 141*t*
   resources for, 182–184
   screening, 26–29, 27*f*
   self-mediated, 141*t*, 149–151, 150*t*
   special education and/or Section
   504 services, 153–155
   teacher-mediated, 141*t*, 143–145
Scientific mindedness, 128–129
Screening procedures, 25–44
   adopted and foster care children,
   130
   common measures used, 28, 28*t*
   for comorbid disorders, 35, 37–39,
   123

DISCARD

Hartness Library
Vermont Technical College
One Main St.
Randolph Center, VT 05061